THE FUTURE FOR HEALTH PROMOTION

Colin Palfrey

T0261684

P

First published in Great Britain in 2018 by

Policy Press
University of Bristol
1-9 Old Park Hill
Bristol BS2 8BB
UK
t: +44 (0)117 954 5940
e: pp-info@bristol.ac.uk
www.policypress.co.uk

North American office:
Policy Press
c/o The University of Chicago Press
1427 East 60th Street
Chicago, IL 60637, USA
t: +1 773 702 7700
f: +1 773-702-9756
e:sales@press.uchicago.edu
www.press.uchicago.edu

British Library Cataloguing in Publication Data
A catalogue record for this book is available from the British Library.

Library of Congress Cataloging-in-Publication Data
A catalog record for this book has been requested.

ISBN 978-1-4473-4123-9 (paperback)
ISBN 978-1-4473-4125-3 (ePub)
ISBN 978-1-4473-4126-0 (Kindle)
ISBN 978-1-4473-4124-6 (ePDF)

Cover design by Robin Hawes
Front cover: image kindly supplied by istock
Printed and bound in Great Britain by CMP, Poole
Policy Press uses environmentally responsible print partners

Contents

List of abbreviations

ACAS	Advisory Conciliation and Arbitration Service
ASH	Action on Smoking and Health
BACP	British Association for Counselling & Psychotherapy
BAME	Black, Asian and minority ethnic
BMI	body mass index
CALM	Campaign Against Living Miserably
CAMHS	Child and Adolescent Mental Health Services
CBR	cost–benefit ratio
CHD	chronic heart disease
EBM	evidence-based medicine
EP	exercise professional
ERS	exercise referral schemes
GP	general practitioner
HSC	Health and Safety Commission
HSE	Health and Safety Executive
IAS	Institute of Alcohol Studies
IHME	Institute for Health Metrics and Evaluation
IMF	International Monetary Fund
LA	local authority
MOH	Medical Officer of Health
NAO	National Audit Office
NCB	National Children's Bureau
NCD	non-communicable diseases
NERS	National Exercise Referral Scheme
NHS	National Health Service
NICE	National Institute for Health and Care Excellence
OCD	obsessive compulsive disorder
PHE	Public Health England
PHW	Public Health Wales
PI	performance indicator
PISA	Programme for International Student Assessment
PPO	Prisons and Probation Ombudsman
QALY	quality-adjusted life year
RCP	Royal College of Physicians
RCT	randomised controlled trial

ROI	return on investment
SMART	specific, measurable, achievable, realistic and time-scaled
TB	tuberculosis
WHA	World Health Assembly
WHO	World Health Organization
WHP	workplace health promotion
YOI	Young Offender Institution

Acknowledgements

My thanks to Ceri J Phillips, Professor of Health Economics at Swansea University, for enabling me to gain access to certain key documents.

I am also grateful to Helen Davis, Shannon Kneis, Phylicia Ulibarri-Eglite and Ruth Wallace of Policy Press for their kindly and efficient assistance during the preparation of the book.

ONE

Main themes

Defining terms

The purpose of this book is to examine the evidence relating to the effectiveness and cost-effectiveness of health promotion policies and projects, specifically but not exclusively in the UK.

First, it is appropriate to clarify, as far as possible, what is generally understood by the key concepts in the health promotion literature. Since this book focuses on health promotion, this phrase needs to be dissected. In addition, definitions – or at least, interpretations of key terms – will be attempted. These include:

- the 'new public health'
- civil society
- poverty
- empowerment

Health

Many commentators would consider dictionary definitions rather bland and inadequate. For example, Chambers (2014) defines health as 'sound physical or mental condition' (p 704), while the *Shorter Oxford English Dictionary* (Little et al, 1933) offers two definitions: 'soundness of body' and 'spiritual, moral or mental soundness' (p.878). None of these three definitions would be acceptable in today's discussions of 'health promotion'. In 1946, the World Health Organization (WHO) referred to 'health' as a state of complete physical, mental and social wellbeing and not merely the absence of disease or infirmity. This has been the prevailing definition up to the present day. There is no mention here of spiritual or moral soundness. These two attributes are more likely to be seen today as the province of religious, humanistic or philosophical/ethical discourses.

An additional dimension to health promotion policy has been an acceptance that factors external to the person's individual

1

lifestyle may have a positive or detrimental impact on their health. This is not a recent acknowledgement; as Chapter Two will show, phenomena such as the quality of air, water supply and rivers became public health concerns well before the 19th century, as did housing conditions and the local environment, and remained concerns into and beyond the Victorian era in the UK. A report by The Health Foundation (2017) viewed health from a social determinants approach, which frames good health in terms of the conditions and attributes that maximise health over the life course and offers a fresh perspective:

> This view would define a 'healthy person' not as someone free from disease but as someone with the opportunity for meaningful work, secure housing, stable relationships, high self-esteem and healthy habits. Understanding health in these terms would highlight lack of employment opportunity and access to affordable housing as a health problem. Rather than simply improving society's ability to respond to disease, more emphasis would be placed on actions that promote the conditions for good health. (The Health Foundation, 2017, p 12)

It can only be assumed that the reference to 'healthy habits' means avoiding certain food, taking enough exercise, avoiding smoking and drinking alcohol (if at all) in moderation. Proponents of health promotion would claim that their concern goes much further than responding to disease, and that there is, in a sense, a tripartite approach to maintaining and improving the health of the nation and individuals. This would involve changing the external factors that damage the 'health' of more economically deprived people, clinical efforts to control and eradicate disease and to treat those experiencing an 'unhealthy' condition, and information and interventions that aim to prevent a lapse into 'ill health'.

What can be extracted from the multiple definitions of 'health', in the context of health promotion, as a guide towards an acceptable and uncontested definition? Perhaps the most logical course is to clarify what health promotion is and is not trying to promote. This will involve seeking authoritative statements on health promotion as a central component of public health policies. Four are listed below.

- Health promotion includes strengthening individuals' skills to encourage healthy behaviours and building healthy social and physical environments to support these behaviours (Health Canada, 2005).
- Health promotion is any combination of health education and related organisational, economic and political interventions designed to facilitate behavioural and environmental changes conducive to health (Green, 1979).
- Health promotion is the process of helping people to take control of their lives so they can choose options that are health giving rather than those that are health risky (Matthews, 1999).
- Health promotion is the process of enabling people to increase control over and improve their health. It moves beyond a focus on individual behaviour and towards a wide range of social and environmental interventions (WHO, 2016b).

Unfortunately, these are not clear definitions of 'health'. However, they imply that health is a desirable condition that depends on a person being able to have control over their lives and not be the subject of external factors that might impair their sense of wellbeing. To return to the initial quest of finding a universally acceptable definition of 'health', we could ask what we mean when we describe a person as 'healthy', or even 'very healthy'. This surely conjures up a vision of someone who is physically active, or even vigorous and mentally alert. It is unlikely that such an individual would remain isolated; therefore, it is highly probable that he or she would also be at ease in company. In short, the WHO's interpretation of the concept 'health' as a state of complete physical, mental and social wellbeing would probably be widely accepted as a useful working definition.

The social determinants of health

Several references will be made in later chapters to the 'social determinants of health'. These have, in some cases, been represented as in opposition to health promotion strategies that aim to improve the health behaviours of individuals and localities (Raphael, 2002). To discover the extent to which health promotion policies, projects and programmes can contribute to a strategy based on the social determinants of health, it is important to identify what constitutes these causes of good and bad health conditions. The WHO set up a commission, chaired by Professor Michael Marmot, to explain how certain sections of the population across the globe suffer much poorer health and have a more limited life expectancy (WHO, 2008). The report, which runs to 256 pages, is concerned with health equity:

> Social justice is a matter of life and death. It affects the way people live, their consequent chance of illness, and their risk of premature death. These inequities in health, avoidable health inequalities, arise because of the circumstances in which people, grow, live, work and age ... The conditions in which people live and die are, in turn, shaped by political, social and economic forces. (p 3)

These inequities are caused by 'the unequal distribution of power, income, goods and services; differing levels of access to health care, schools, education, conditions of work and leisure, their homes and chances of leading a flourishing life' (p 9). These factors prompted the commission to recommend a number of actions to offset or, more optimistically, close the health gap within a generation. These are:

1 improve daily living conditions, including early child development;
2 place health equity at the heart of urban governance and planning;

3 ensure that economic and social policy responses to climate change and its environmental degradation take into account health inequity;
4 ensure fair employment and permanent, decent work that pays a fair level of income, and avoid poor working conditions and stress;
5 build healthcare systems based on the principles of equity, disease prevention and health promotion;
6 proper regulation of goods and services that have a major impact on health, such as tobacco, alcohol and food;
7 reduce unequal levels of pay for men and women.

To underline the serious gaps in health and life prospects, the report provides some illustrative statistics:

* The prevalence of long-term disabilities among European men aged 80 and over is 58.8% among the lower educated versus 40.2% among the higher educated.
* Over 80% of deaths from cardiovascular diseases occur in low- and middle-income countries.
* Of people with diabetes, 80% live in low-and middle-income countries.
* The lifetime risk of maternal death is one in eight in Afghanistan; it is one in 17,400 in Sweden.
* Maternal mortality is three to four times higher among the poor in Indonesia compared with the rich.

It is clear from the WHO commission's seven aforementioned areas for action that reducing gaps in income and the physical environment in which people live are outside the province of health promotion. Within the UK, the Black Report (1980) recorded marked differences in mortality rates between the occupational classes, for both sexes and at all ages. It noted that, at birth and in the first month of life, twice as many babies of unskilled-manual parents die as do babies of professional-class parents, and in the subsequent 12 months four times as many girls and five times as many boys will die. A class gradient was observed for most causes of death, which was particularly steep in cases relating to the respiratory system. In addition, self-reported rates of longstanding illness were twice as high among unskilled-manual males and 21 times as high among working class women as among their counterparts in the professional classes.

Nearly two decades later, the Acheson (1998) report on inequalities in health found that inequalities by socioeconomic group, ethnic group and gender could be demonstrated across a wide range of measures – and that the differences between those at the top and those at the bottom had widened. The report recommended that the government seek to influence some of the wider determinants of health, such as employment; income; housing; transport, education and the benefits system.

Neither of these UK reports mentions the potential of health promotion initiatives to address the social determinants of health. This is not unexpected, since the term 'social determinants' only partially defines the broader influence on health, such as government policies. The means to abandon the necessity of food banks, sleeping rough and reliance on benefits is within the purview of the government of the day. In this context, health promotion must be the responsibility of those who wield political power, with only limited opportunities for those employed in the health service.

The new public health

Chapter Two will devote much of its content to describing early attempts to combat the spread of noxious diseases that affected large sections of the UK population throughout the nineteenth century. Because of the widespread disease pattern, the health of the public on a national scale became a concern of the government. How and why a government reacts to epidemics prompts a fundamental question of motive. It is apparent that during the Victorian period of outbreaks – such as cholera, typhoid, tuberculosis and influenza – the impact on the economic and military standing of Britain in the world encouraged governments to take action. Today, although some previously controlled maladies such as tuberculosis and pneumonia are on the increase, they are not present on an epidemic scale. Those that are – such as obesity, diabetes and dementia – pose a challenge to governments in the UK, which are largely looking to public health to ease the problem. This in turn leads to a need to rationalise the allocation of resources on the basis of the main reason for interventions, such as health promotion projects. Are attempts to improve people's health prompted by a desire to reduce absenteeism and so preserve a high rate of productivity, or a commitment to the ethical imperative that good health is a human right, or the need to control rising expenditure on the National Health Service (NHS) – or perhaps all three?

During the course of the 20th century, advances in clinical treatments and medical technology put paid to many diseases. However, during the 1970s, conventional medicine came under attack from two sources (Mold and Berridge, 2013). First, the rising cost of healthcare made high-tech medicine increasingly expensive. Second, some influential studies, notably those reported on by McKeown at the University of Birmingham, argued that declining mortality rates at the end of the 19th century were not so much the result of medical advances but of improved living standards and nutrition (McKeown, 1979). Although McKeown's thesis was criticised as doing little justice to the positive impact on the nation's health through the interventions of modern medicine, much greater reliance was placed on health promotion as a preventative – and therefore more cost-effective – health strategy. As a crucial element of the UK's developing public health strategy in the 1990s, health promotion as a model of health policy has become accepted from all political perspectives (Hann, 2000).

Civil society

This is a name that appears in many formal reports on health policies (WHO, 2007; IMF (2017). Civil society refers to collective action around shared interests, purposes and values. It includes charities; nongovernmental organisations (NGOs); community groups; women's organisations; faith-based organisations; professional organisations; trade unions; social movements, coalitions and advocacy groups. There is no one 'civil society view', but despite its complexity and heterogeneity, the inclusion of civil society voices is essential in giving expression to the marginalised and those who are not often heard (WHO, 2007). According to Laverack (2014), civil society is the totality of voluntary, civic and social organisations that together form the basis of a functioning society. It is important because it stresses the need for a developed level of public and political participation, both central to health promotion. Civil society organisations have to use a variety of tactics to achieve their goals and achieve more political influence. They occupy the space between governments and business organisations.

The WHO (2008) emphasised that the continued involvement of civil society, and the participation of communities in work on social determinants of health, will be fundamental to chances of succeeding in closing the health inequalities gap in a generation.

What is 'poverty'?

For decades, ill health and poverty have been associated as cause and effect, where either has been seen as cause or effect. As such, it is important to try to define, or at least describe, what we mean by the term 'poverty'. In *Hamlet*, the theme of madness – feigned or otherwise – pervades the play. On hearing that Hamlet appears to be mad, Polonius, the wise old Lord Chamberlain, offers this observation: 'For to define true madness, what is't but to be nothing else but mad' (Act 2; scene 2). In similar tautological terms, the dictionary definition of 'poverty' is 'the state of being poor' (Chambers, 2014). Even in Victorian times, very few families could have been accurately described as being in a state of 'destitution', which implies a lack of life's necessities such as a roof over one's head, food and family or social support. Interestingly, attitudes towards the poor have changed little over the centuries and largely depend on varying definitions. The *pauper* addressed in the Elizabethan Poor Law 1601, which consolidated four previous Acts, was someone who had no income and had to rely on charity to survive. But a distinction was made between the deserving and the undeserving poor; a distinction that in essence has survived into our own times.

The Act for the relief of the Poor, popularly known as the Elizabethan Poor Law 1601 categorised the 'deserving' as the elderly, the very young and the infirm, while pickpockets, highwaymen, migrant workers and beggars were categorised as 'undeserving'. In Victorian times, some social commentators believed (with little hard evidence to support their views) that many poor families were in that state because of a lack of 'thrift', as some mothers and fathers wasted money on alcohol (Fitzpatrick, 2001). Today, there are people on benefits who would no doubt be regarded as deserving of state support, while others would merit the title of 'skivers'. In the UK, there are proponents of health promotion who blame poverty for the unhealthy diets of people living in areas of relative deprivation – a term offered in some quarters as a synonym for 'poverty' (Townsend et al., 1988). Others challenge this as a probably unfounded assumption based on little or no empirical evidence (Bennett and Murphy, 2001).

In Victorian times, there were soup kitchens; today, there are food banks. But who exactly are the 'poor'? The official political definition is that a family existing on less than 60% of the median income of the population is deemed to be 'in poverty' – a definition that could be open to criticism. Basically, it could be argued that all averages – whether mean, median or mode – can be misleading. Fairly recently, the number of units of alcohol that health experts state should not be exceeded has reduced from 21 to 14 for men – the same as that specified for women. This takes no account of a person's height, weight, rate of metabolism or whether they are drinking on an empty stomach or with/after a meal. Interestingly, in the 1990s, the safe level for men was set at 50 units, and 35 for women (Baggott, 2000). Similarly, the medically determined 'ideal' blood pressure has varied over time.

The problem with a relative definition of poverty is that, like alcohol and blood pressure measures, the definition is likely to alter – partly because of more informed medical diktats, but also because of changing social circumstances. Let us suppose that, in 10 years' time, the median income in the UK increased to £100,000 per annum. Applying the same relative comparison, any family whose income fell below £60,000 per annum would be considered to be 'in poverty'.

The impact of public health and health promotion interventions

There is compelling evidence that the Public Health Act 1875 improved the nation's state of health. Sanitary authorities were established with a responsibility for sewerage, water supply and refuse disposal, and between 1850 and 1900 average life expectancy increased by 10 years. Again, the 'average' cloaked the disparity in levels of health between the social classes; people in the 'lower classes' experienced shorter lifespans than the more affluent sections of the population.

Today, no such dramatic improvements as a result of public health initiatives can be easily recognised. For example, Wanless (2004, p 18), contended that 'the major constraint to further progress on the implementation of public health interventions is the weakness of the evidence base'. Similarly, McQueen and Jones (2010, p 35) argued that: 'The reality of health promotion practice is that causality is almost always too complex to describe with much degree of probability, let alone determination'. When we add the comments of Berridge (2010, p 22): 'Historical evaluation of health promotion ... cannot tell us what works best, what is cost-effective ... or advise us on the best technique for assessment' and Naidoo (2010, p 108): 'Currently policy decisions are being made with only limited experimental knowledge on [sic] the effect of interventions', the prospect of acquiring tangible proof of the value and efficacy of health promotion policy and projects appears somewhat remote. Much of the debate about a deficiency of evidence centres on the key issue of evaluation methodology – a topic that will feature in Chapter Three.

In addition, the question of differing targets and objectives of health promotion and health education needs to be raised. If, for example, it is accepted that relatively poor health is mainly due to socioeconomic factors that characterise particular communities, then efforts should be made to improve family incomes through enhanced job opportunities and improved benefit levels. However, Green and Thorogood (1998) have argued that health promotion alone is unlikely to have any significant impact on socioeconomic factors. For this reason, perhaps, many advocates of health promotion have directed their efforts towards changing people's lifestyles and behaviour. Yet this approach has its detractors. Breslow (1990), for example, notes that the main drawbacks of a strategy that emphasises individual action and personal choice are that:

• It ignores the social context in which individual choices are made, and so cannot tackle the wider influences on health; that is, it runs the risk of 'blaming the victim'.
• A community approach is preferable in creating social and environmental conditions that would be more conducive to health.

Dixey et al. (2012) probe even more fundamental ethical issues relating to the development of strategies designed to improve people's health. They put the case for people's right to privacy, and question whether there is any justification for interfering in people's lives through 'social engineering', persuasion and encouraging or even coercing people to behave in certain ways – a view that Aldermann (2013) supports. The authors refer to Ewles and Simnett's (2003) questioning of who has the right to say that an 'unhealthy' lifestyle is 'wrong'. It is important to note that 'health is not the only consideration in people's lives' (Dixey et al., 2012, p 90).

Today, the internet, social media and articles in newspapers and magazines contain ample information about how to live a healthier lifestyle. Indeed, it could be argued that there is almost an obsession with the need to avoid certain foods, take more exercise and reduce alcohol intake to minimise the risk of succumbing to heart disease, strokes and cancer. So, apart from specific planned interventions from government (both national and local), what impact is the spread of information having on improving the health of the population – or, at least, certain sections of the population? Le Fanu (1994, p 16) is in no doubt that health education 'takes the form of advertising slogans – or rather admonitions – which, were they complied with, are presumed to improve the health of the nation: don't drink and drive; wear a condom; smoking kills; eat healthily etc.'. He continues: 'scientific attempts to evaluate health education promotions almost all show that it is actually very difficult to get people to change their behaviour by cajoling them to do so' (p 90).

However, as Cragg et al. (2013) have pointed out, even if health promotion measures have an effect, it is likely that the effects can only be recorded over a long period and will be difficult to measure. This raises the question of 'intervening variables'; that is, while there may appear to be a correlation between a certain health promotion or health education initiative, any discernible impact on lifestyle or improved health might be the result of some other factor – such as a move to a healthier environment or housing, a school campaign to encourage pupils to eat healthier food and/or take part in sporting activities or a local authority's decision to provide free leisure centre activities during off-peak hours – all of which could be quite distinct from the government's health promotion project(s).

What is the purpose of health promotion?

This would seem to be a rather naive question, since it resembles the tautological nature of attempts to define 'poverty'. The purpose of health promotion is surely to promote health. But dictionary definitions of the verb 'to promote' are not very helpful – although 'to raise to a higher level' probably comes close to the interpretation of 'health promotion' as an attempt to raise the level of people's health. Interestingly, the term 'promotion' also carries the meaning of 'advertising' – of 'selling' an idea to the public.

One of advocates' key targets for raising the levels of people's health is the increasing incidence of obesity. Yet, despite media coverage of obesity as an increasing phenomenon, adults and children do not appear to be heeding warnings about the potentially harmful effects of being very or extremely overweight.

Haslam et al. (2014, p 214) state that 'despite numerous ... government initiatives there is still a significant section of society that seems ... unwilling to accept basic health messages that obesity, including that in childhood, is bad for health'. In the same vein, Green and Thorogood (1998) make the point that a psychological approach to health promotion seeks to answer why, despite everything they know about its health hazards, some people still eat sugar. One answer to this could be that people who eat sugar in various forms are prepared to ignore the possibility of future damage to health in favour of the immediate satisfaction of a taste they particularly like. The disregard of health warnings could be attributed to at least three causes:

• People may be unconvinced that the evidence for the negative effect of certain 'behaviours' is sufficiently cogent.
• People do not take kindly to what they regard as another facet of the 'nanny state'.
• People's eating habits are largely determined by their social and economic circumstances.

A relevant framework for addressing people's noncompliance with government health warnings is the dual questions of (a) whether this behaviour is deliberate or unavoidable, and (b) why a government would wish to prevent or delay illness in the general population.

We have already noted the lack of evidence about the effectiveness of health promotion initiatives. One obvious gap is the dearth of empirical studies gathering evidence from people living in areas of relative deprivation about their lifestyle, including the types of food they eat; whether they take any exercise; their intake of alcohol; whether they smoke – all constituents of what 'experts' claim have a recognisable influence on health or ill health. One conclusion, founded on scant or even absence of hard evidence, is that people whose diet is considered to be undesirable cannot afford to buy healthier food. This is debatable because there is no data available to give us a reliable picture of the dietary preferences of those considered to be economically disadvantaged. Do they, for example, prefer to buy relatively expensive takeaway or instant meals rather than buy ingredients to make cheaper and presumably healthier food? It would be difficult to blame lack of exercise on poverty in the 21st century, since even those living in high-rise flats or substandard housing could take exercise that is free of charge, such as walking. Of course, critics of the 'blame the victim' approach to health strategies would claim that much of the problem of unhealthy lifestyles is due to stress and a range of mental health problems. This will be discussed in Chapter Six.

A key landmark in health promotion was the publication of the document *The Health of the Nation* (Department of Health, 1992). This focused on six health problems: coronary heart disease; stroke; cancer; mental illness; HIV/AIDS and sexual health, and accidents. These were chosen because they were deemed to be major causes of premature death or avoidable ill health in which effective interventions should be possible. The strategy also identified a number of settings, such as schools, homes and the workplace. However, criticisms of the document included that it failed to tackle the social and economic factors that had a bearing on poor health, that it followed a medical and epidemiological model of health and that it ignored phenomena such as poverty, inequality, stress and housing conditions. These were social and environmental factors beyond the scope of the NHS, the responsibility for which lay with central and local government (Baldock et al., 1999). Proponents of the case for governments to go well beyond a determination to change unhealthy lifestyles and to concentrate on alleviating distressing and morale-sapping external conditions would contend that attempts to 'educate' individuals and communities are ineffectual and patronising.

This must raise the question of why any government would want to invest in health promotion and health education. If some people actually choose to indulge in a lifestyle that carries with it a 'health warning', what right has anyone to try to change their behaviour? Even in the face of evidence that poor diet, lack of exercise, exceeding the recommended limits on alcohol consumption and smoking are detrimental to health, adults can often cite examples of certain people – sometimes famous people – who have lived to a grand old age despite what would be regarded as an unhealthy lifestyle. Winston Churchill, for example, who died at the age of 91, was devoted to his cigars and brandy and claimed – though this might be apocryphal – that the only exercise he got was helping to carry the coffins of friends who took exercise. Of course, relatively isolated examples of longevity being personally attributed to the opposite of a healthy regimen do not necessarily undermine the evidence of what leads to avoidable morbidity and premature death.

However, the ever-rising incidence of childhood obesity in the UK and many other countries is a cause for concern about responsible parenting. There have been instances in which children have been taken into care because of their parents' inability or unwillingness to prevent them becoming unhealthily overweight (Johnston, 2014). The prospect of future generations of children becoming prone to illnesses that could have been prevented by a healthier upbringing quite naturally prompts those in authority to have regard for children's welfare – but to what purpose?

Motives for improving people's health

Empowerment

Empowerment has been defined as a process by which people, organisations and communities gain mastery over their affairs (Rappaport, 1987). In the context of health promotion, 'affairs' relates to individuals gaining control over their health and collective action to address social injustice. The WHO defines health promotion as 'the process of enabling people to increase control over and to improve their health' (WHO, 2009a, p 1). This process involves helping people to develop the skills they need to make healthy choices (Ashton and Seymour, 1988).

This would appear to be a laudable motive for assisting less-informed individuals and communities to achieve a similar set of values to those of the more informed, more educated social strata. Yet it must be asked whether there is permissible scope for the objects of health education and health promotion to make unhealthy choices. Is 'empowerment' in itself a choice, or is this strategy in effect an imposition? Green and Thorogood (1998, p 47) suggest that 'Self-empowerment ... is really about making "middle-class" skills and experience available to the culturally impoverished ... working class'.

There is also the question of *how* individuals and communities can be empowered. One route could be the role of health education in giving people the appropriate knowledge about what a healthy lifestyle entails: which foods to avoid and which to eat; what body mass index (BMI) is and how it can signify a dangerous level of body fat; how binge drinking can lead to serious health problems. As noted earlier, there is such a preponderance of information about 'healthy choices' in the media that it would seem unrealistic to suppose that a certain section of society is unaware of potentially harmful lifestyles. So, is it socially acceptable to still smoke cigarettes, to eat mainly fast food and takeaways and/or to make no effort to reduce one's weight?

Tones draws attention to the possible limitations of the self-empowerment model of health promotion: 'For those seeking to promote self-empowerment, the capacity to freely choose is success enough even if an individual should choose not to reduce the risk of coronary heart disease' (Tones, 1986, p 11). This could be interpreted as something of an ironic statement, since the purpose of much health promotion activity is to deter people from making wrong choices. But who is to assess what is meant by 'wrong'? Wrong in what sense, and in what circumstances? If, for example, it can be proved that social isolation, unemployment and reliance on benefits contribute to relatively poor health, a successful attempt on behalf of governments and public bodies would be required to remove these impediments to health and wellbeing. Without such economic improvements, a healthy choice would be severely restricted.

As an alternative scenario, what if an individual had no such restrictions and decided to ignore health warnings and advice? Is this 'wrong'? Is it 'irrational'? Can an unhealthy lifestyle be seen as an example of self-harm? Those in authority who strive to promote a philosophy of empowerment would be very uneasy about accepting the alternative rationality of grown adults who are prepared to put pleasure before risk aversion. Can anyone be condemned for harming themselves if by doing so they inflict no harm on anyone else?

Charity

The dictionary definition of 'charity' is 'the disposition to think favourably of others and to do them good' (Chambers Dictionary, 2014, p 264). Certainly, this attitude of compassion proved the starting point for the earliest attempts to reduce the morbidity and mortality rates of the poor in the 17th century. Three centuries later, the Second World War had a profound effect on nurturing a degree of political unity towards issues of social divisions in terms of standards of living and standards of health between the haves and have-nots. During the war, there was a coalition government of the Conservatives and Labour. One of its primary aims was not only to ensure 'a home fit for heroes' (which Prime Minister David Lloyd George proclaimed during the previous world war to be a fundamental right of all returning service personnel) but also to cater for the much broader social and economic needs of the population. Towards this end, the government commissioned the Liberal William Beveridge to produce a report, the eventual title of which was *Social Insurance and Allied Services*, which was published in November 1942. The result was the formation of a welfare state.

The report identified what became known as the 'five giants': squalor, ignorance, disease, want and idleness. The symbolism of a knight riding out to defeat these monsters had no resonances of Don Quixote's tilting at windmills; these giants were not illusory, but all too real. As far as disease was concerned, the response was not immediate because of some cross-party concerns about the economic consequences of such far-reaching reforms. However, in 1944, the Conservative Minister of Health, Henry Willink, was responsible for a White Paper that would provide the foundations of the NHS. The White Paper proposed no less than the creation of a fully comprehensive, universal healthcare system, free of charge and available to all citizens, irrespective of their means.

However, voters at the general election on 5 July 1945 returned a Labour government, two months after Germany surrendered and exactly 12 months to the day after the National Health Service Act became law. The incoming health minister was Aneurin Bevan, a fervent left-wing socialist, who described the Tories as vermin. Nevertheless, he fully accepted the contents of the White Paper and emphasised his unflinching commitment to enable access to a state-funded and state-run health service for everyone. He wrote that no society can legitimately call itself civilised if a sick person is denied medical aid because of lack of means (Bevan, 1952).

In a sense, the NHS introduced what could be called 'state charity'. The Act was designed to help people who were unable to help themselves, and this policy in itself was built on the beliefs that everyone wished to enjoy good health and that good health should be a right, not a privilege for the relatively well-to-do. This incontestable principle was enshrined in the health education and health promotion initiatives that took root in the UK in the 1980s under the banner of the 'new public health'. A detailed analysis of the main impetus for health promotion will feature in Chapter Four.

Economics

Following the institution of the NHS in July 1948, government assumed that, with free treatment for all, the scale of illness in the population would decrease. As a result, the cost of providing services would in turn also decline. An alternative logic might have predicted that quite the opposite would happen. The cost of ever-more complex medical technology has soared; the numbers of people living into advanced old age have risen dramatically, putting pressure on hospital and community services; and people's expectations of care when they are ill have substantially increased (Baldock et al., 1999). As a result, the prospect of financing the NHS throughout the UK has become a major economic and political challenge.

Policies to counteract or at least minimise costs have tended to focus on diverting services away from hospitals and into the community, with a strong emphasis on expanding services offered by primary care (Department of Health, 2006). Attempts have also been made to persuade people to think twice before calling on ambulance services to transport them to a hospital when their perceived health problem could more appropriately be dealt with elsewhere and with much lower costs (Snow, 2007; Edwards, 2014). A key aspiration of those who strenuously support a strategy of health promotion – namely, that it will not only help towards sustaining and improving the nation's state of health and wellbeing but also reduce costs – is probably ill-founded (Phillips, 1997).

This assertion has been made most tellingly in the field of mental health (which will feature in Chapter Six), in which early intervention focusing on preventing mental health problems is considered to accrue considerable cost savings. Such savings have been calculated in relation to lost productivity, amounts spent on benefits and the costs of replacing workers who leave their jobs because of mental ill health (Friedli and Parsonage, 2009). These calculations, however, have been challenged. Le Fanu (1994), for example, has argued that the resources used on health promotion would be better spent on treating the sick than preventing people becoming ill. This would appear to question the very foundation and rationale of the new public health: that 'prevention is better than cure' because it is cheaper.

Those who query the value of a preventative approach to dealing with the health of the nation do so on the grounds that there is insufficient evidence that health promotion works, and that if indeed it *does* have a positive effect, such an impact can only be measured over a long period of time. Therefore, efforts to estimate its cost–effectiveness and/or its cost–benefit might be sabotaged by intervening variables, so that prevention of disease or reduced levels of mortality could be attributed to alternative factors – such as access to employment and increased income and, as a consequence, a reduction in stress. Surprisingly, one of the reasons why the evaluation of health promotion and health education initiatives has proved difficult is the lack of community-based research in which local residents have actually been asked whether such initiatives have had any influence on their lifestyles over a particular period of time.

Evaluation

Methods for evaluating the results of health promotion initiatives are a crucial concern of policy makers and practitioners. In May 1998, the World Health Organization (WHO) urged all member states to 'adopt an evidence-based approach to health promotion policy and practice, using the full range of quantitative and qualitative methodologies' (WHO, 1998b). However, this has proved difficult to accomplish in terms of gathering 'evidence' that is uncontroversially valid. As noted earlier in this chapter, Wanless (2004, p 18) (for one) has drawn attention to the inherent flaw in attempts to produce convincing data: 'the major constraint to further progress on the implementation of public health interventions is the weakness of the evidence base', while Killoran and Kelly (2010, p 35) have commented that: 'The reality of health promotion practice is almost always too complex to describe with much degree of probability, let alone determination'.

To move from a *correlation* between a health promotion programme and an improved state of health and wellbeing to *causality* is often problematic, not least because of the lengthy timeframe within which such a programme has to operate. For example, Davey and Popay (1993) claimed that evaluating the effectiveness of disease prevention could mean a randomised controlled trial (RCT) involving about 30,000 people over a period of 10 years. The RCT, sometimes referred to as the 'gold standard' for evaluating the effect of healthcare interventions, relies on the ability to compare at least two relatively large groups of people with highly comparable characteristics – such as age, gender and social class – and introducing a particular input to one group and no input (or a placebo) to the other. The validity of the ensuing data will rely on the extent to which the groups have been protected from any other so-called 'intervening variables' invading the experiment.

Clearly, over an extended period of time, the capacity of experimenters (or health promotion implementers) to insulate the intended beneficiaries from factors other than those identified as the health promotion components is likely to be compromised. For this reason, qualitative methods for evaluation, rather than RCTs, have been proposed (Scott, 2001). Such methods could include the use of focus groups and/or individual interviews, self-complete questionnaires, participant observation, journals kept by participants and official documents (Davies and Macdonald, 1998).

Community

Reference has already been made to the concept of 'empowerment' as a particular concern and objective of health promotion advocates. It is all too easy to use benign-sounding terminology without strictly defining terms. For example, it could be argued that the words 'sustainable' and 'robust' have become so overused in official documents and policy statements that they have become what might be described as 'apple pie' notion; that is to say, they are examples of linguistic laziness because they serve as synonyms for anything that could be termed 'acceptable' or 'desirable'. In the same way, it might be tempting to refer to 'community' as a cornerstone of health promotion policy without clearly articulating what its essential quality really is. What, for example, is meant by 'community engagement'? Laverack (2009, p 10), for example, states that 'health promotion aims at complementary social and political actions, such as advocacy and community development' without explaining what 'community development' actually entails. Laverack does, however, list the 'key characteristics of "community"'. These are:

- a spatial dimension (a place or abode);
- nonspatial dimensions (interests, issues, identities) that involve people who otherwise make up heterogeneous and disparate groups;
- social interactions that are dynamic and bind people into relationships with one another;
- identification of shared needs and concerns that can be achieved through a process of collective action.

A much earlier definition anticipated Laverack's attributes of both shared interests and space. The Calouste Gulbenkian Foundation (1984) referred to a grouping of people who share a common purpose, interest or need in some particular geographic locality. The UK government's document *Our Healthier Nation* (Department of Health, 1999) was not content to regard a community in relatively neutral terms; instead, it extended the definition to one of a *healthy* community, which was typified by characteristics such as acceptance of diversity, mutual respect, high-quality public services and good transport links (Department of Health, 1999).

The future for health promotion

The concluding chapter of this book discusses the crucial issue of the future for health promotion. Doubts about the worthiness of health promotion initiatives – and particularly about the cost-effectiveness of schemes to prevent ill health and/or improve the level of health and wellbeing in areas of economic disadvantage –demand close investigation as to their source. There is also some debate about the ethical acceptability of the methods chosen to launch and monitor health promotion projects. For example, while slogans such as 'empowerment', 'reducing health inequalities' and 'the fair distribution of resources' feature strongly in the literature, some commentators consider these undeniably worthy causes to be innately top-down and therefore disempowering (Davey and Popay, 1993; Green and Thorogood, 1998).

As noted at the beginning of this chapter, even more fundamental is the potentially disputed assumption that 'health' is an unequivocal concept. The United Nations definition of a state of complete physical and mental wellbeing has been criticised for ignoring a person's spiritual or emotional health (Dines and Cribb, 1993). Dines and Cribb (1993, p 13) maintain that 'it would be more useful to emphasise the dynamic nature of health rather than see it as a state which is relatively unchanging'.

Another area of disagreement is whether efforts to persuade people to adopt healthier lifestyles are:

1 of any use, because the main cause of relatively poor health is determined by the individual's social class, income and physical environment;
2 unethical, because they are an assault on people's freedom to adopt the lifestyles they prefer;
3 essentially attempts by the middle classes to impose their values and priorities on those who do not share their relative affluence and chosen lifestyle.

Dines and Cribb (1993, p 42) are clear exponents of (1) and (2); they maintain that: 'If individuals do not always give the pursuit of health absolute priority then it is far from obvious that the State or health professionals should do so on their behalf'. As far as point (1) is concerned, Chapter Four will provide substantial evidence that this view is held by a large corpus of health promotion advocates. It could be argued, then, that the future for health promotion will depend largely on the evidence base for adopting one or another of the strategies laid out in various government policies, both within the UK and elsewhere.

TWO

The origins of health promotion

Diseases in Britain before and during the 19th century

Public health becomes the concern of governments when disease becomes widespread and when there are good grounds for believing that something can be done about it. In Britain, as in many other countries, epidemics have a history of causing death on a huge scale. Between 1348 and 1350, the Great Pestilence, which became known in the 17th century as the Black Death, killed an estimated 40–60% of the population of England (Campbell, 1991). This pestilence returned in 1361, and again in the 15th century. Unfortunately, there was no known cause other than the wrath of God for sin or the disastrous conjunction of planets. London was the worst affected part of England, but the disease spread to other areas including Bristol and Cumbria, and the plague eventually engulfed most of the country. It was only several centuries after its first appearance that the cause was identified as bacteria from fleas carried by rats.

This information, which would come to be known as the aetiology of disease, heralded the beginnings of a public health movement, which gained momentum throughout the 19th century. At this time cholera was the most prevalent life-threatening disease, but others gained much more than just a foothold (Harris et al., 2012). Typhus – caused by bacteria transmitted to humans via parasites such as lice, fleas and ticks – was rampant in English prisons, where men were crowded together in dark and filthy rooms in which lice could spread easily. The complaint started in Ireland but crossed to England after a short while. Cholera and typhus were not the only pervading diseases in the 19th century; smallpox and tuberculosis were also responsible for thousands of deaths. Smallpox is caused by viruses and tuberculosis by airborne bacteria transmitted by coughs and sneezes.

Shortly after the traumas of the Second World War in Britain had subsided, the government turned its attention to a form of health education through its propaganda cinema film entitled *Coughs and sneezes spread diseases* (British Pathé, 1947). The threat of tuberculosis had not been eliminated. This short film, which portrayed a middle-aged man being shown the way to reduce the spread of disease by means of using a handkerchief every time he anticipated sneezing, was a prime example of a public health message that stressed personal responsibility as one way of avoiding unnecessary harm to others. The combination of public health measures to improve environmental conditions and a call for personal attention to healthier living became a hallmark of government strategy as the 19th century progressed.

Public health in the 19th century

It is perhaps not widely known that Florence Nightingale was a very prominent campaigner for a programme in Britain of what we now know as public health. Her modest aspiration – that the very first requirement of a hospital was to do the sick no harm – was motivated by a realisation that medical interventions were not proving to be an effective remedy for many serious illnesses, especially epidemic diseases (Small, 1998). Her work as a nurse in India during the uprising in 1857 and during the Boer War that began in 1899 convinced her that bad drainage, contaminated water, overcrowding and poor ventilation were causing the high death rate.

Having become highly proficient in the collection and analysis of statistical data, she reported that, after 10 years of sanitary reform, mortality from diseases among soldiers in India had declined from 69 to 18 per 1,000 (Cohen, 1984). On returning to Britain, she was active in urging the government to adopt a more radical and far-reaching policy in its attempts to improve the health and living conditions of the population. She lobbied the minister, James Stansfield, to strengthen the proposed Public Health Bill to require property owners to pay for connection to mains drainage. This requirement became included in the public health acts of 1874 and 1875 (McDonald, 2004).

During the Victorian era, the spread of cholera caused huge public concern – even though other diseases such as typhus, smallpox, scarlet fever and tuberculosis caused more deaths (Logan, 1950). The peak of deaths from cholera came in the years 1848–49, with over 53,000 deaths in England and Wales (Creighton, 1965). Firm evidence of the cause of this and other diseases was not forthcoming, but the root of the problem was assumed to lie in filthy living conditions as towns became more heavily populated. The Public Health Act 1848 allowed localities outside London to establish health boards, the responsibilities of which included managing sanitation and waste disposal. Much of the impetus for the creation of this Act came not from politicians but pressure groups, notably the Health of Towns Association (Hollis, 1974).

In contrast, the medical profession did not wholeheartedly support the public health movement during its early phases. More influential was Edwin Chadwick, secretary of the Poor Law Commission and secretary to the Health of Towns Association. He and other reformers (such as Sir John Simon, who sat with Chadwick on the General Board of Health) faced opposition from organisations with vested interests to protect – notably the water companies, which resisted the additional expenditure that sanitary reforms would incur, and industries that regarded measures to impose a quarantine on goods imported from foreign countries as injurious to their livelihoods.

The Poor Law Amendment Act 1834

As one of the architects of this law, which laid down the principle that only the most destitute should receive assistance, Edwin Chadwick applied Jeremy Bentham's (1789) philosophy that the success of any enterprise should be measured according to whether it secured the greatest happiness of the greatest number. The full title of the Act was The Poor Law Amendment Act because it revised the previous Act of 1601. It followed a number of acts in the 16th century and clearly defined different categories of poor people. These were:

- the *impotent poor* (such as physically disabled, visually impaired and elderly people), who were genuinely unable to work and were to be cared for by the parish in almshouses or poorhouses;
- the *able-bodied poor*, who were set to work in a House of Industry;
- the *idle poor, vagrants and beggars*, who were sent to a house of correction or even prison;
- *children*, who would be helped to become apprentices.

In essence, therefore, two types of relief were to be administered: indoor and outdoor. This discriminatory provision between the deserving and undeserving poor involved finding work in a strict indoor environment or allocating money, food or clothing for those considered worthy of assistance from the parish. Why the government at the time considered it necessary to help the poor will occupy part of Chapter Seven, which raises a similar question about current welfare and health policies in contemporary Britain and elsewhere.

The provisions of indoor and outdoor relief continued in England and Wales under the 1834 legislation. Although the Act did not directly address the problem of poor people's ill health and weak resistance against infectious diseases, it prompted the Poor Law Commission to appoint three doctors in 1838 to study the possible link between illness and poverty. The doctors – Kay, Southwood Smith and Arnott – investigated conditions affecting public health in London. These and further investigations culminated in Chadwick's (1842) report, *The Sanitary Condition of the Labouring Population of Great Britain*. Perhaps even more persuasive in highlighting at least a correlation between environmental conditions and sickness was the statistical evidence produced by William Farr, a statistician with a medical background. His research showed the health disparity between residents of poorer areas and those of more affluent parts. His contribution to the establishment in Britain of a more scientific approach to discovering and dealing with the causes of disease, especially epidemics, deserves a special mention.

The Poor Law Amendment Act was implemented unevenly across England and Wales. More importantly, the diet of people assigned to the workhouses was deemed inadequate to sustain their health. Charles Dickens's novel *Oliver Twist* captured the criticisms levelled at this situation from workers, politicians and religious leaders.

William Farr (1807–83)

William Farr was a pioneer in the field of epidemiology. His appointment in 1838 to the General Register Office – the government department for recording births, marriages and deaths – spurred him on to set up a system that recorded the *cause* of death. Edwin Chadwick, who admired Farr's work, strongly supported this innovation. One of Farr's most interesting (if contested by some) analyses arose from the cholera epidemic in 1849. He concluded that the miasma – foul vapours and air caused by rotting matter – had a more deleterious effect on the health of people who lived in low-lying ground along the banks of the River Thames, which was heavily polluted with sewage, compared with those on higher ground further away from the river.

This finding was not widely disputed at the time, but the clear linkage demonstrated by John Snow between the next cholera outbreak and a particular water source – the Broad Street pump – persuaded Farr that water rather than air was the more likely cause of disease transmission (Halliday, 2000). However, it must not be assumed that the rather tenuous link between foul air and disease and illness in the case of the cholera outbreak discredits the possibility of airborne elements leading to health problems, or even death. Current concerns about the impact of air pollution caused by industry and motor vehicles will feature in Chapter Eight's discussion of contemporary public health issues.

Such public health issues as inequalities in the health status of residents in poor and affluent areas were already forming an important part of Farr's research. In an analysis of the 1837 death records, he attributed 63 deaths to starvation (Farr, 1839). This finding caused considerable concern in government circles, since it was assumed that the Poor Law Amendment Act 1834 guaranteed sufficient sustenance even for workhouse inmates and those receiving outdoor relief. In addition, he mapped out what he termed 'healthy districts', and compared mortality rates between those and unhealthy districts. In one of his many annual letters to the Registrar General in which he reported on his analyses of the latest mortality statistics, Farr calculated that from 1851–60, 65,000 children's lives were lost in the unhealthy districts (Farr, 1864).

Of course, to produce such statistics is only a preliminary contribution to any relevant action that a government could or should take to diminish the extent of health inequalities. The next crucial stage is to identify the cause(s) of such disparities. If it can be proved that 'poverty', however defined, leads directly to starvation or the inability to pay for preventative or curative treatment, then a government or its delegated authorities should be able to take the appropriate action.

The Public Health Act 1848

In 1842, Edwin Chadwick published *The Sanitary Condition of the Labouring Population of Great Britain* at his own expense, as the Poor Law Commission did not want to be associated with the report. However, it need not be assumed that Chadwick's concern stemmed wholly from a deep-seated philanthropic motive. Indeed, the Poor Law Amendment Act itself was based on the principle that its criteria for assistance would largely deter people from seeking relief, especially given the prevailing conditions in the workhouses. One of Chadwick's key arguments was that improving the health of the poor would result in fewer people seeking poor relief; this, in turn, would save money.

The Act's provisions centred on improved drainage and provision of sewers, the removal of all refuse from houses and streets, the provision of clean drinking water and the appointment of a medical officer for each town. After campaigning by the Health of Towns Association and another severe outbreak of cholera in 1848, a previously reluctant government yielded and the Act of 1848 became law. The Act established a central Board of Health, but this had limited powers and no funding. Loans, however, could be taken out for developing more hygienic environments, and the money paid back from the rates. Where the death rate was higher than 23 per 1,000, local boards of health had to be set up (Baggott, 2000). After the Act of 1848, the Health of Towns Association was disbanded and other groups became active in the public health campaigns, notably the Social Science Association and the Sanitary Institute (Hollis, 1974).

Disputes about the causes of ill health and early deaths were persistent in the 19th century. Proponents of sanitary reform could not accept the proposition that poverty was the main cause of ill health in Britain. After all, this was a period of expanding industrialisation. Yet this phenomenon created its own health problems. By attracting potential workers into towns, this increasing urbanisation too often led to overcrowding and housing inadequate to accommodate sizeable families. What the poor needed, according to many observers, was not 'relief' but a more responsible approach to maintaining their health. They needed education (Kelly and Symonds, 2003). What policy makers needed was clear and indisputable evidence about the primary causes of diseases and epidemics so that these health problems could be treated and hopefully eradicated.

Resistance to state intervention

Efforts to improve the environment in which people lived and worked were the dominant form of attempting to deal with public health, while advances in medical science were relatively slow. Ironically, the introduction of vaccinations in Britain after Edward Jenner's successful treatment of smallpox in 1796 caused stern public resistance. The main issue was the introduction in 1853 of compulsory vaccination of smallpox sufferers. Widespread local campaigns made it difficult to enforce the law (Baggott, 2000). The main reason for such opposition was that compulsion was an assault on individual liberty. When the General Board of Health was disbanded in 1854 as a result of public pressure, its demise was greeted with enthusiastic approval in *The Times*: 'The British nation abhors absolute power. We prefer to take our chance with cholera and the rest than be bullied into health' (Longmate, 1966, p 188). This resistance to what some regarded as state interference in personal choices about attitudes to the threat of disease has resonances with the views of some much more recent commentators on public health policies. Reference has already been made in Chapter One to what today would be termed 'the nanny state', and there will be further discussion on this issue in succeeding chapters.

In 2017, *The Times* reported on parents' opposition to having their children vaccinated against flu. This arose partly from a flawed research report in which a former doctor linked vaccines with autism (Loy, 2017). Because there has been no compulsion for children to be vaccinated, the rate of vaccinations has dropped over the past few years. Apart from anxiety about the possible side effects of the vaccination, which is administered to young children via a nasal spray, parents quoted in *The Times* report cited the objection that yearly vaccinations could overload their children's immune system and that the vaccine had not been sufficiently tested to convince parents that it was safe.

One of the most articulate advocates of civil liberties in the face of central control was John Stuart Mill (1806–73), who was at odds with what came to be known as 'utilitarianism' – the creed of Bentham and his supporters. Interestingly, Bentham had a marked influence on Mill's early education, but he later rejected Bentham's philosophy. In 1848, he wrote *Principles of Political Economy*, in which he argued that governments should sacrifice economic growth for the sake of the environment and that the population should be limited, in accordance with the work of Malthus (1798), to avoid the risk of starvation for the overburdened poor.

Even more relevant to the views of succeeding politicians in the UK, Mill argued that individual liberty should be the cornerstone of governmental policies. His *Essay on Liberty* (1860) emphasised his belief that the only purpose for which power can be rightfully exercised over any individual against their will is to prevent harm to others. The individual's own good, whether physical or moral, was not a sufficient reason. He accepted that efforts could legitimately be made to persuade someone to do what was considered 'right', but argued there should be no compulsion. This approach sent a clear message – still relevant today – that there should be agreed limits to the role of governments, and society in general, in trying to shape human behaviour (Cragg et al., 2013).

The Public Health Act 1875

The Public Health Act 1875 represented the culmination of the sanitary reform movement. It consolidated previous legislation relating to public health made during the 19th century. The Act established an obligation on local authorities to provide clean water, dispose of sewage and refuse and ensure that only safe food was sold. It gave them the power to do what Florence Nightingale had campaigned for: to ensure that existing and new homes were connected to the main sewage system. The Local Government Board was given the power to prevent the spread of diseases such as cholera, and for two or more local authorities to work together to prevent or reduce the spread of epidemics. As Baggott (2000) has remarked, this Act set a framework for the next 50 years in public health.

These powers were very similar to those imposed by the previous Act of 1848. An additional power accorded to local authorities was to inspect for 'nuisances', for which they could serve abatement notices. A 'nuisance' could be cumulative deposits of refuse, overcrowding in homes or unclean workplaces.

Public health towards the end of the 19th century has been described as an admixture of benevolent despotism, ratepayers' self-interest and social control (O'Keefe et al., 1992). There was a gradual move away from the call for sanitary improvements to the need for preventative medicine (Wear, 1992). As an increasing number of local authorities appointed medical officers of health (MOH), the influence of individuals with a medical background began to grow. MOH began to exert influence at both local and national levels. They formed their own separate organisation in 1856 and helped to draft public health legislation, as did the British Medical Association (Bartrip, 1996). However, the 'sanitarians' – such as Sir John Simon, who was appointed as the Medical Officer to the Board of Health in 1855 – continued to identify social and environmental conditions as the main causes of afflictions such as cholera, diphtheria and tuberculosis.

Despite this lingering adherence to sanitary improvements, the status of the medical profession was gradually enhanced, particularly through studious research in the spheres of epidemiology and bacteriology. Snow's aforementioned discovery of an unequivocal causal link between cholera and the drinking of polluted water served to disprove untested hypotheses about the damaging effect of miasma from the sewage-infested River Thames. However, this did not demolish contemporary moves to improve sanitation, as there were other diseases whose origin was not definitely known. In 1864, Louis Pasteur promoted his germ theory; but 100 years before, a Scottish surgeon to the Royal Navy worked on and published his scientific enquiries into the cause or causes of scurvy, which was rampant among the crew of ships (Lind, 1753). He had assumed that scurvy was probably the result of a number of factors, but eventually came to the well-founded conclusion that citrus fruit would be a successful antidote to the disease.

Yet it was only with what might be termed the 'bacterial revolution' of the 1880s that the scientific discoveries of Snow and Lind came to be fully appreciated and accepted. The emphasis now was on preventative medicine, not just improving living conditions in towns. Wear (1992) and Lewis (1992) have pointed out that, towards the end of the 19th century, the laboratory became the focal point for epidemiological research. The laboratory also emphasised the importance of medical interventions that could be more easily measured than social interventions. The problems inherent in evaluating the impact of health education and health promotion initiatives among targeted populations will be discussed in later chapters. While the capacity of modern medicine to cure some previously prevalent and persistent diseases has been a major stepping stone towards the health of the nation, attempts by governments to reduce the incidence of mortality rates caused by unhealthy lifestyles have proved frustratingly ineffective.

Naturally, the sheer complexity of public health as a national issue meant that a medical focus on the individual did not negate the need to ensure that populations were not exposed to social conditions such as poverty and related environmental problems, including unclean air. Today, just as new viruses can overturn advances in the treatment of illnesses such as cancer, so the side effects of industry can have a negative impact on the atmosphere of big conurbations and lead to a global concern to reduce the prospect of global warming.

Monitoring and surveillance

Green and Thorogood (1998) noted that the shift from sanitary reform to a more scientific model of public health demonstrated a shift from a lay to a medical perspective. The prevention of ill health became a medical activity requiring the skill of doctors, and one which now focused on individuals' behaviours rather than the conditions in which they lived (Baggott, 2000). Nevertheless, it was recognised that disease, if not always of epidemic proportions, was endemic in Britain. The nature and degree of such diseases will be discussed later in this chapter. For whatever reasons – humanitarian, economic or a combination – the government believed it was its own responsibility to monitor the situation and make every effort to control it.

With the increase in population during the latter half of the 19th century, the need to intervene in people's lives was seen as essential to maintain what might be classified as 'social order'. It is perhaps difficult, living in a post-NHS society, to appreciate the dire circumstances in which many sick parents and families lived. Paying for healthcare during a period when the medical model of healthcare became the norm was out of the question for huge swathes of the population. Some element of compulsion had to be accepted by both citizens and relevant organisations if the general health of the population was to be monitored and improved. In 1870, for example, the Compulsory Education Act brought about a nationwide inspection of schoolchildren's teeth.

Nettleton (1992) has described the development of public health practice from the 19th century onwards as moving from a wholly environmental approach (sewers, drains, housing) to the epidemiological phase with child health surveillance and the 'dispensary'. It became important, as it is today, to try to understand why people persist in what are considered to be unhealthy behaviours. Health education became an important component of health policy. The third phase placed individuals in their socioeconomic and cultural context as a means of understanding why some indulged in what might be described as 'self-harm'. However, as Baggott (2000) has pointed out, it would be wrong to interpret the emphasis on individuals and subgroups as entirely new. Much of the impetus for the sanitary movement arose from studies into the conditions of the poor. In addition, personal hygiene had long been an important focus of campaigns to control disease.

The coexistence of the personal and the public is not unique to 19th-century efforts to stamp out large pockets of unacceptably low levels of health. As noted in the previous chapter, the sometimes-uneasy twin government strategies of accepting that people with relatively poor health are the victims of poverty on the one hand, and attempting to persuade individuals to eat more healthy food, abstain from smoking cigarettes, reduce the intake of alcohol and take exercise on the other, are present today.

This duality of government strategies was most clearly exemplified in the 19th century by the local sanitary associations, which employed 'visitors' to provide advice and education on health matters. For them, personal hygiene was as important to combating disease as improvements in clean streets and houses. However, there was mounting pressure for the state to tackle poverty and destitution. According to Wohl (1984), public health reformers in the Victorian era failed to address in any concerted manner the prevailing environmental and economic inequalities across social classes. The possibility of this apparent reluctance might in part be attributed to a traditional religious acceptance that this was what God had ordained. After all, the Sunday school hymn *All things bright and beautiful*, which was published in 1848 (a seemingly crucial date in the chronology of public health movements), contained the lines: 'The rich man in his castle; the poor man at his gate / God made them high or lowly and ordered their estate'. This third verse has been expunged from any recital of the hymn, but it was not until 1982 that the London Education Authority banned it (Christiansen, 2007). This tacit acceptance of the gaps within the social hierarchy was perhaps an unspoken attachment to the status quo.

Whatever the predominant reason, many of the 'sanitarians' who had sought to break the cycle of poverty and disease experienced a high degree of frustration. This was notably so for Sir John Simon, who fully acknowledged the role of poverty in leading to disease; in his role as medical officer, he described poverty as among the worst of sanitary evils. However, as Webster (1990) and Honigsbaum (1970) asserted, the Local

Government Board's Poor Law functions tended to overshadow any radical move towards real social reform. Poor Law officers were mainly concerned with providing care for the poor, but after the creation of the Local Government Board in 1871, the functions of the Poor Law and sanitation were brought under its aegis. Yet instead of exercising a close integration of both functions, the gulf between public health and the Poor Law widened after this date (Hodgkinson, 1967).

Summary of legislation

It would be helpful at this point to list the relevant legislation enacted during the 19th century in Britain, and then to concentrate in more detail on the concept that so dominated the work of Chadwick – poverty.

1832   Reform Act (Poor Law Commission with Chadwick as Secretary)

1836   Registrar General established (first recording of population statistics)

1842   Chadwick's *Report on The Sanitary Condition of the Labouring Population of Great Britain*, which led to the rise of the sanitary movement

1848   First Public Health Act
        Appointment of Sir John Simon as Medical Officer of Health

1866   Sanitary Act: placed local authorities under the obligation to inspect their district

1868   Housing Act: local authorities could ensure that owners kept properties in good repair

1871   Local Government Board Act (became Ministry of Health in 1919)

1872   Public Health Act: made appointment of a Medical Officer of Health compulsory

1875   Public Health Act: increased powers of local authorities and brought together all aspects of public health law. Local authorities to establish their own sanitaria

One of the impediments to a truly national public health service was that, at an early stage in the legislation, much of it was advisory or permissive rather than compulsory. As a result, some of the worst environmental hazards in the lives of poor families and individuals were not necessarily addressed and alleviated by the responsible authorities. Furthermore, some of the statistical data on which action was based caused one social reformer to carry out a painstaking empirical survey of the poor in Britain. This person was Charles Booth (1840–1916).

Charles Booth and poverty in the late 19th century

When campaigning on behalf of the Liberal Party in 1865 in Liverpool (his hometown), Booth was appalled by the squalid living conditions in the slums. This experience confirmed in him an enduring sense of obligation towards the poor. The success of the Tory party in the succeeding election disillusioned Booth regarding the likely impact of politics on ameliorating the lot of deprived citizens. In 1884, having moved to London, he assisted in analysing census returns for the appropriate allocation of the Lord Mayor of London's Relief Fund. He was not satisfied that the census depicted the true nature of poverty in the city, and resolved to check whether his discomfort with both the scope and accuracy of the figures would be confirmed by organising his own more meticulous social audit. With the help of his wife Mary and a number of other helpers (including Beatrice Webb, a socialist reformer who worked with her husband Sydney in the Fabian Society and helped to found the cooperative movement), Charles Booth set out to gather information under three sections: poverty, industry and religious influence. The results of the survey were published in 1903 (Booth, 1903).

One of his sources of data was the school boards, which provided details of pupils' parents' poverty levels and types of occupation. The industry component investigated virtually every trade in London and the wages and conditions of employment. The series of searches also covered the 'unoccupied classes', inmates of institutions (primarily the workhouses) and causes of pauperism. The religious influences focused more on people's moral stances and the impact of these on their ability to cope with everyday living. By 1899, descriptive, colour-coded maps of different areas of London were published to show the varying levels of poverty throughout the city. The worst areas were covered in black. The concluding volume in the series was published in 1903.

During the last decade of the 19th century Booth served on a number of bodies, including the Royal Commission on the Aged Poor (1893) and the Royal Commission on the Poor Law (1907, with Beatrice Webb). His studies persuaded him that the impoverished older generation was in need of more than charity and good works. What they needed was some financial security, however limited this might be. He therefore agitated for a universal old-age pension, and the Liberal government of the day passed the Old Age Pensions Act in 1908, which introduced a means-tested rather than universal pension.

Booth's political sympathies were far from socialist. He did not readily assume that poor people were not responsible for their own and their family's poverty. His main motivation for his comprehensive survey of life among the poor in London was to avoid unproved assumptions and replace them with facts. Hence his insistence on not only asking third parties such as the school boards for whatever details they kept on pupils' parents but also walking the streets of London himself and visiting houses. For example, whereas there was a belief that poverty existed, but in limited numbers, Booth's findings showed that 30% of London's population were living in poverty (Fried and Elman, 1971).

Booth also visited the homeless, who lived in fairly squalid lodging houses or on the streets – a situation that has not disappeared in Britain today. His main interpretation of his empirical data was that poor people were not in every case personally responsible for their situation, but that their impoverished incomes prevented them from obtaining acceptably hygienic housing conditions or affording accommodation that was not grossly overcrowded. Booth defined the 'poverty line' as a level of means required to avoid starvation. This definition, of course, has been considerably modified in the context of life in 21st-century Britain.

Seebohm Rowntree (1871–1954)

Benjamin Seebohm Rowntree was born in York. He shared Booth's view that most impoverished people were likely to fall into poverty for reasons beyond their control rather than their own moral failings. His first study of poverty in York was published in 1899, his second in 1935 and his third in 1951. He and his investigators visited over 11,500 working-class homes in the city and discovered that 27.84% were living below what he described as the 'poverty line', a percentage highly comparable to the results in Booth's survey. His research was more explicitly tied to the relationship between poverty and ill health than Booth's surveys. He classified the poverty line as a sufficient income to enable a family to secure the necessaries to enjoy a healthy life (Coates and Silburn, 1970). For this purpose, he consulted contemporary nutritionists to discover the minimum calorific intake to prevent a person losing weight and becoming susceptible to sometimes serious illness. The results were published in *Poverty: A study of town life* (Rowntree, 1901).

The money needed for this basic subsistence level covered fuel; light; rent; food, clothing and essential household items. One very interesting (and officially unacknowledged) finding was that those in old age or early childhood were the most likely to be in abject poverty, so he formulated the idea of the 'poverty cycle' that some people might move in and out of during the course of their lives (Searle, 2004). Rowntree's unique contribution to the study of poverty and health was his conclusion that, according to his more liberal description of the necessities of life (which included newspapers, books, tobacco, holidays and presents), poverty was now the result of unemployment and not low wages. This is not surprising in view of the nation's plight during the period of economic depression towards the end of the 19th century (Musson, 1959).

His third survey, published in 1951, portrayed a Britain in the climate of 'the affluent society'. Some pockets of absolute poverty remained – for example, among the elderly – but it was assumed that this lingering problem would be solved through the nation's access to welfare benefits. Rowntree proved to be somewhat ahead of his times in recommending family allowances and a minimum wage. From 1907, he was influential in his role as an adviser to David Lloyd George towards creating the Old Age Pensions Act 1908 and the National Insurance Act 1911. Lloyd George was Chancellor of the Exchequer from 1908–15.

The Boer Wars and public health

The wars between the Boers (South African farmers) and Britain lasted from 1899 to 1902. It shocked the government that 60% of potential recruits to the army were considered unfit for service. This prompted not a humanitarian concern but a fear that Great Britain (with an emphasis on 'Great') could be overtaken economically by its main rivals: Germany and the US. The scale of poverty revealed by Booth and Rowntree was accepted as having a clear impact on the nation's health. If men of military age were unfit for service, the government was worried about Britain's ability to defend itself against a strong enemy, especially an increasingly militaristic Germany. If Britain was to remain a powerful industrial and military force in the world, then the health of its children and young people had to improve.

As a result, the government set up a committee to focus on the physical condition of the population. In 1904, its findings were published. It recommended improvements in the standard of food and drink; regulations to avoid overcrowding and air pollution; the training of schoolgirls in cookery and hygiene; the provision of meals for underfed children and medical inspections in schools. The dominant war cry became 'national efficiency', as the country became aware that Germany had implemented a host of social welfare policies that included sickness and accident insurance and old-age pensions. This convinced leading thinkers and politicians that 'national efficiency' in Germany relied substantially on ensuring its people were physically and mentally healthy.

As a result, the timely survey results promoted by Booth and Rowntree, together with the stark analysis of Boer War statistics on the proportion of unfit recruits, influenced the Liberal government to introduce the two significant aforementioned acts: for old-age pensions and a system of National Insurance. The strategy for improving the nation's health had shifted to an extent: from concerns with and action on unhealthy living environments, to a willingness to help vulnerable people – young and old – to climb out of poverty in order to reach a level of health that would not only give hope and some security to the poor but also provide the basis for an increasingly invigorated workforce. These legislative provisions were instrumental in preparing Britain's defensive capabilities as it began to arm itself for the First World War (Winter, 1980).

Key legislation in the 20th century prior to the establishment of the NHS

The recognition during the last decade of the 19th century that Britain's economic future lay with the younger generation propelled the Liberal government to bring in legislation to ensure children would grow up healthy and physically fit. For this reason, school became the focal point of appropriate legislation. In addition, the surveys carried out by Booth and Rowntree proved that not all poor people were idle, that many who were in employment were paid low wages, and that if the worker was ill the money would stop. The days of the Poor Law 1601, which made people avoid the penal conditions of the workhouse at all costs, were well and truly over. Despite his acceptably humane motives, Chadwick was nevertheless keenly committed to deterring people from being idle rather than rewarding the industrious.

Key pieces of legislation in the 20th century (prior to the establishment of the NHS) were as follows:

1902   Midwives Act: licensed midwives now employed by local authorities under the supervision of the MOH

1906   Education (Provision of Meals) Act: school meals

1907   Education (Administration) Act: began the School Medical Service
        Notification of Births Act: provided for the employment of health visitors

1908   Old Age Pensions Act: provided a weekly pension for those aged 70 and over

1911   National Insurance Act: when the worker was ill,
        money was paid for a limited period of time
1918   Maternity and Child Welfare Act: local authorities
        made responsible for routine health check-ups of
        children
1929   Local Government Act: transferred some hospitals
        into direct local authority control
1936   Public Health Act: consolidated the public health
        functions to be provided by local authorities
1942   Beveridge Report: identified the 'five giants' that
        had to be destroyed: want, disease, ignorance,
        squalor and idleness.

The National Insurance Act 1911 was, at least in part, a political
move to offset the inroads being made by the recently formed
Labour Party. The Liberal government was eager to send a
message to the working classes that they cared about their welfare.
But there were not to be any free handouts if the worker lost
employment because of illness. Employers, employees and the
state were each to contribute towards a fund, which would
provide an income if the individual became ill and unable to
work for more than three days, and gave the worker free access to
medical treatment to enable them to return to work as quickly as
possible. This Act was compulsory, and so was fully implemented.
However, the Act of 1906 was voluntary, with the result that
many local authorities took no action. Neither was the Act of
1918, which introduced medical inspections of schoolchildren,
made compulsory; although these inspections were free, any
resulting need for treatment had to be paid for. This left many
children assessed as in need of medical intervention without
treatment because their parents could not afford it (Gazely, 2003).

Booth and Rowntree had shown that a great deal of poverty
was due to old age. Both New Zealand and Germany had
enacted pensions legislation two years prior to Britain's Act of
1908. Just two years after a resounding electoral victory in 1906,
the Liberal Party began to lose a number of by-elections to the
Labour Party. It was therefore imperative to be seen to be on
the side of the poor and to make old-age pensions provision
compulsory. No contribution was necessary. The funds were

to be paid for out of taxation, and paid through post offices to avoid the stigma of the Poor Law. However, the Act of 1908 excluded those in receipt of poor relief, those in 'lunatic asylums', those who had been sent to prison 10 years after their release, persons convicted of drunkenness and anyone found guilty of habitual failure to work (Macnicol, 1998). On the positive side, the pension was available for men and women, provided their yearly income did not exceed £31.10 shillings.

The Act was only a partial success. While it did indeed keep many out of poverty, the amount of the pension was below the calculated poverty line. Furthermore, at the start of the 20th century, the minimum age of 70 at which a pension could be claimed was significantly above the average lifespan, particularly that of relatively poor people. There was also a restriction on who could claim; if a person had claimed via the Poor Law in the previous 10 years, they would not be allowed to claim a pension.

Prior to the National Insurance Act, other legislation aimed to protect workers from penury if they became ill or injured. The Workmen's Compensation Act 1906 attempted for the first time to deal with unemployment on a national scale. Local authorities could form distress committees. Work was provided where possible, and from now on, unemployment – with its links to poverty and ill health – became a national responsibility.

The Beveridge Report 1942

William Beveridge, a young civil servant, made a close study of unemployment and had been greatly impressed with German labour exchanges (Cootes, 1967). By this means, the unemployed could be made aware of any vacancies that existed. As a result of his efforts to convince the government of the need for labour exchanges in Britain, 83 such facilities were opened in Britain in early 1910. But not every corner of Britain subscribed to the government's efforts to intervene in the lives of those who were poor or threatened with poverty if they became out of work. For example, many in the medical profession opposed the National Insurance Act 1911, foreseeing the beginnings of a national health service – which, at its inception in the National Health Service Act 1946, was indeed opposed by doctors. They argued that if such a service were to be created, they should run it. Their opposition, as in the run-up to the NHS, was overcome by offering them attractive financial opportunities and conditions. Winston Churchill described the National Insurance Bill as the most decisive step on the path towards social organisation. He stressed its importance by declaring that 'the cruel waste of disease and unemployment, breaking down men and women, breaking up homes and families, will for the first time be encountered by the whole strength of the nation' (Cootes, 1967).

Although social insurance was extended to workers outside the key industries referred to in the Act of 1911, the period of economic depression in the 1920s and 1930s put increasing pressure on the government to devise a comprehensive system. In 1941, a committee of inquiry was set up to undertake a survey of existing national schemes of social insurance and to make recommendations. By this time, William Beveridge had become established as a prominent and highly respected civil servant and academic, and he was appointed chairman of the committee. His report was published in 1942 to public acclaim, although the government had not promised to adopt any recommendations, merely to consider them. Among the recommendations to tackle the 'five giants' was the proposal to establish a truly national health service, through which everyone – irrespective of financial means – could obtain free medical treatment. This would be financed via general taxation, with a small element contributed from the National Insurance scheme, which would be comprehensive in its coverage and to which everyone in employment would have to contribute. Attendance at doctors' surgeries and hospitals was free, as were medicines prescribed by the doctor (which could be collected from dispensing chemists), eye tests and spectacles from the optician and dental treatment. The National Health Service Act became law in 1946.

Public health and the media

In the middle of the 20th century, the diseases that had dominated the public health agenda in the previous century were no longer the main concern of the British government; a new scare was created by the exhaustive research findings of Richard Doll and his colleagues. Much of his research concentrated on the causes of different cancers, and in 1950 he co-authored an article in the *British Medical Journal* that proved a causal link between cigarette smoking and cancer of the lung (Doll and Hill, 1950). At first, political reaction was to play down the seriousness of this research result, since it was felt that a panic reaction would put a strain on NHS resources. In addition, the government was absorbing a considerable tranche of tax revenue from the tobacco companies.

The public health strategy had moved from sanitary measures to reducing the prevalence of diseases to offsetting the health-related problems brought on by poverty. The new public health of the 1950s and 1960s tended more towards encouraging personal responsibility for safeguarding individual health. Smoking was not a disease but a health risk; ultimately, demands on the health service through rising levels of cancers in the population had to be addressed.

For this reason, a public awareness campaign was launched (in which television played an increasingly important role) to not only persuade smokers to quit or take up the less harmful forms of cigar and pipe smoking but also avoid drinking alcohol and driving. An influential report was produced by the Royal College of Physicians in 1962 (RCP, 1962), which drew on research data to spell out in great detail the health hazards of smoking. The RCP pointed out that continuing smoking would lead to a high risk of contracting lung cancer, bronchitis and heart disease. At the time of the report's publication, the RCP reported that 75% of men and 50% of women were smokers. The Central Council for Health Education and local authorities spent £5,000 on antismoking advertising in 1956–60, while the tobacco industry spent £38 million on promoting their products (Berridge and Loughlin, 2005).

The RCP recommended a public education campaign through advertising. The authors wanted restrictions on the sale of tobacco to children under 16 (a policy that was being ignored by too many shopkeepers), a restriction on cigarette adverts and a ban on smoking in public places. In the same year as the report's publication, the Institute for Health Promotion and

Education was formed. With devastating diseases on an epidemic scale now overcome by medical advances, health strategy turned towards educating the public on the risks of unhealthy lifestyles and behaviours. In 1964, the Cohen Committee of the Central and Scottish Health Service Councils also recommended a national advertising campaign against smoking, and in the 1970s this coverage was transmitted through television. Another development was the formation of Action on Smoking and Health (ASH) in 1971 by the Royal College of Physicians. ASH is a charity that works to reduce the burden of addiction, disease and death attributable to tobacco.

Throughout the 1970s, the 'new public health' began to place much more emphasis on personal responsibility but, as the Secretary of State for Social Services pointed out in a speech to the National Council on Alcoholism, it seemed difficult to modify social attitudes and to measure what effect (if any) had been achieved (Ministry of Health, 1981). By the 1980s, the notion of 'health promotion' began to replace that of health education. Health promotion was about encouraging 'positive health' and preventing illness rather than curing it. However, it did not neglect earlier policies of working with communities to develop healthy environments and efforts to explore the relationship between poverty and ill health (Mold and Berridge, 2013).

The New Public Health

In the 1970s, the Labour government sought to raise the profile of prevention and health promotion issues by publishing the consultative document *Prevention and Health: Everybody's Business* (DHSS, 1976). This identified key areas for future intervention: heart disease; road accidents; smoking-related diseases; alcoholism; mental illness; drugs, diet and venereal disease (Baggott, 2000). Its orientation towards prevention was strengthened by some influential reports from the World Health Organization. The *Declaration of Alma Ata* (1978) followed by the *Global strategy for health for all by the year 2000* (1981) clearly stated that health is a fundamental human right and that health policies should be pre-emptive and precautionary, the aim being to prevent the problems from arising at the earliest possible stage.

to mean a lasting concession, and not one that is capable of being revoked when a parliament so decrees.

The other salient question is: empowerment for what? Ashton and Seymour (1988) observe that health promotion works through community action: 'At the heart of this process are communities having their own power and having control of their own initiatives and activities' (p 26). They go on to state that health promotion aims to help people develop the skills they need to make healthy choices. However, this objective can be challenged from three different perspectives. First of all, how does a 'community' cope with the health hazard of air pollution? A vigorous campaign to challenge an offending industrial plant's activities or reduce the noxious gases caused by diesel-powered traffic might be successful. But this is not an example of being *given* power; it is an example of people *taking* power. Second, the concept of 'the right choice' or 'the healthy choice' could be regarded as disempowering. Propaganda to stop people smoking in the 1950s and 1960s elicited some responses claiming that smoking comforted people and relieved stress. In effect, the very concept of 'health' propagated by those in power appeared to ignore a sense of mental wellbeing.

A third objection to what might be seen as a hazy notion of empowerment is the argument that forces beyond the control of individuals and communities limit their opportunity to follow a 'healthy' lifestyle. The fact that poverty is still regarded in Britain today as an impediment to free choice highlights the need for governments at local and national levels to take the appropriate action. Communities in the more economically deprived areas of Britain are experiencing poorer states of health, and subsequently higher mortality rates, than residents living in the more affluent areas (Black Report, 1980; Laverack, 2014). The answer, it might be argued, is not empowerment but enhanced employment opportunities. Thus, critics of the conventional health education and health promotion models maintain that: 'Any attempt, therefore, to educate people to make informed health choices in such [constrained] circumstances is not only ineffective but unethical' (Tones, 1986, p 8). It is unethical, according to some commentators, because it is really about trying to engender middle-class values among the socially impoverished working class (Green and Thorogood, 1998).

Black Report 1980

In August 1980, the UK Department of Health and Social Security published the report of the Working Group on Inequalities in Health, known as the Black Report after its chairperson Sir Douglas Black, President of the Royal College of Physicians. The Labour government commissioned the report in 1977. The report concluded that, many years since the establishment of the welfare state and NHS, there had been very little progress in reducing health inequalities in Britain. The morbidity and mortality rates differed significantly between the different occupational classes; in fact, these inequalities had been widening. However, the report did not consider that this was because of a failing NHS. It laid the blame on other causes, such as inadequate incomes and poor housing, diet, unemployment and working conditions.

In 1979, a Conservative government had been returned to office, and the report's findings were disregarded when the report saw the light of day in 1980. The then Secretary of State declared that the cost of taking the recommended actions would be prohibitive and that there was no firm evidence that such actions would have the desired effect. In the next decade, several research-based statistics confirmed the Black Report's findings and indicated a disturbing trend in different mortality rates between the top and bottom socioeconomic strata of the population (Blane et al., 1990; Phillimore et al., 1994; Drever and Bunting, 1997).

The Thatcher and Major Conservative governments were reluctant to acknowledge the existence of health inequalities, or at least that they were caused by poverty. In their view, such class differences in health status were down to the fact that the manual classes indulged in unhealthy activities by choice. It was not up to the government to try to eliminate or reduce inequalities in income. It was the role of the NHS to help when people became ill (Baggott, 2004). This approach was encapsulated in a Department of Health report in 1995 with the title *Variations in health: What can the Department of Health and the NHS do?* (Department of Health, 1995). The report drew criticism from the medical profession. They deeply regretted that its authors failed to consider issues such as housing, unemployment, poverty and job insecurities, which many saw as the underlying causes of health inequalities (Wilkinson, 1996).

Health promotion and the social determinants of health

Future chapters in this book will examine the evidence for statements about (a) the causes of ill health; (b) the impact of attempts to tackle these causes; and (c) the quality of health promotion research. On this last point, a report from independent UK charity The Health Foundation called for improved research methods to generate valid data about both (a) and (b) (Health Foundation, 2017). The report followed a social determinants line, setting out its priorities for national policy action to change perceptions from ill health to positive health. Its fundamental ideology is that people's health is influenced by political, social, economic, environmental and cultural factors. With more space to develop this contention, it would be helpful to offer examples of each determinant's influence. The report goes on to state that 'health is not just about wealth' and to cite statistics showing that, despite its superior national wealth, the US experiences lower life expectancy than France, Sweden, Spain, the UK and Japan, and although the US spends more on healthcare than the UK it has a higher prevalence of heart disease, diabetes and cancers (ONS,2016). It will be important in succeeding chapters to try to determine the reason for these differences.

Concluding thoughts

The history of what might be termed the 'public health movement' has been characterised by a tension between the 'environmentalists' and those who sought to alter people's habits. Yet this is a false dichotomy. There are good grounds for attributing continuing differences in health status between more and less affluent areas to *both* causes. While most economically advanced countries have cast off the shackles of prevalent and fatal diseases, there remain health problems in the 21st century that could claim the label 'epidemic'. One of these is obesity, particularly child obesity. Another is drug abuse. And while the benefits of cleaner cities and medical advances have contributed to an ageing population, this same positive outcome has brought its own attendant crisis in the ability of the NHS to respond to increasing demands for care and treatment.

The key question is: How can an emphasis on health promotion impact on health problems brought on by forces outside the control of the individual or the physical environment in which they live? From another standpoint: How can health promotion strategies persuade people to adopt a healthier lifestyle if (a) it is in fact their environment, living conditions and low income that have led to their unhealthy choices; or (b) they have the means to live a risk-free life but choose not to do so?

To answer these questions, it is necessary to examine the evidence that underpins differing attitudes towards reducing health inequalities, and the means by which such evidence has been obtained. This is the subject of the next chapter.

THREE

Evidence base and methods for evaluation

How do we know that health promotion is having an impact on preventing ill health, improving health status and reducing health inequalities? At this point it is worth reiterating two references from Chapter One:

> The major constraint to further progress on the implementation of public health interventions is the weakness of the evidence base. (Wanless, 2004)

> In May 1998 the World Health Assembly urged all Member States to 'adopt an evidence-based approach to health promotion policy and practice using the full range of quantitative and qualitative methodologies'. (WHO, 1998b)

With a plethora of criticisms about the seemingly innate problem of discovering whether health education and health promotion interventions are effective, it becomes questionable whether investment in such projects is justifiable. Yet the commitment to health promotion as a worthwhile preventative strategy remains a central element in the repertoire of healthcare systems in the UK and abroad. However, if these criticisms have any validity, how might they be countered?

Berridge (2010) appears to point the way to a significantly different methodological approach to evaluating the effectiveness of health promotion in action: 'Historical evaluation of health promotion ... cannot tell us what works best, what is cost-effective ... or advise us on the best technique for assessment' (p 22); 'Health promotion needs to establish methodological rigour and scientific credibility if it is to achieve recognition as a discipline' (p 30).

The question of developing an evidence-based discipline in the context of health matters has not been confined to health education and health promotion. It has been preceded by a debate about the benefits of evidence-based medical practice. Cochrane's (1972) innovative methodology was inspired by what was seen as the fallibility of the medical profession in forecasting, with any degree of accuracy, the probable impact of their treatment on a patient's health and wellbeing. Cochrane was an early exponent of a much more rigorous method of testing the efficacy of clinical interventions. He promoted the need for randomised controlled trials (RCTs), in which experimental and control groups are used so that the key variable – treatment of some kind – can be isolated and checked for its effect (Palfrey, 2000). However, this scientific approach did not convince everyone concerned with medical interventions. Fowler (1997), for example, dismissed it as something of a slur against medical professionals' judgement and a sure means of rejecting or delaying medical advances.

Fowler's (1997) rather acerbic rejection of the whole notion of evidence-based medicine (EBM) regarded it merely as a synonym for informed decision-making. 'The presumption is made', wrote Fowler, 'that the practice of medicine was previously based on a direct communication with God or by tossing a coin' (p 242). Equally dismissive and sardonic was Greenhalgh's view that EBM is:

> The increasingly fashionable tendency of a group of young, confident and highly numerate medical academics to belittle the performance of experienced clinicians by using a combination of epidemiological jargon and statistical sleight of hand ... the argument, usually presented with near evangelistical zeal, that no health-related action should ever be taken by a doctor, nurse, a purchaser of health services or a politician unless and until the results of several large and expensive research trials have appeared in print and been approved by a committee of experts. (Greenhalgh, 1997 pp 3–4)

One of the problems of adopting only one method of evaluation, such as the RCT, is that it ignores other methods that might have equal validity. Sackett et al. (1996) argued that 'without clinical expertise, practice risks becoming tyrannised by evidence, for even excellent external evidence may be inapplicable to or inappropriate for an individual patient' (p 71). Clearly, in the health promotion field, conducting RCTs could prove to be extremely challenging – a claim that will be examined further in Chapter Eight. For example, many projects take place over months, or even years, in which case it is likely to be logistically impossible to retain exactly the same cohorts of subjects in the 'experimental' and 'control' groups. For this reason, other evaluation research methods will need to be tried. These are discussed later in this chapter, and in the final chapter of this book.

One of the main weaknesses of health promotion policy is that its objectives are often unmeasurable. An early example, which was applied to the NHS as a whole, was the Merrison Report of 1979 that arose from the Royal Commission's deliberations on the NHS. In this report, the objectives that the NHS could be expected to achieve were as follows:

• to encourage and assist individuals to remain healthy;
• to ensure equal entitlement to services;
• to provide a broad range of services of a high standard;
• to ensure equal access to these services;
• to provide healthcare free at point of use;
• to satisfy reasonable public expectations for healthcare;
• to provide a national service responsive to local needs.
(Merrison Report, 1979)

The difficulty here is that these objectives do not include any timescales and are not specific enough to enable evaluators to judge whether or not they had been achieved. A similar problem prevails today because so many policy statements relating to health promotion are vague (as noted in Chapter One). There will be further discussion of some of these statements, but at this point it is important to flag up some key objectives, such as empowerment, community involvement, equality and health itself. It will also be relevant to analyse (a) the different constituents of formal evaluation (input, process, output, outcome and impact), and (b) to identify the criteria by which each of these may be tested.

Performance indicators (PIs)

Weiss (1972) made a relatively early attempt to define evaluation, which she referred to as 'judging merit against some yardstick' (p 1). This definition refers only to the *process* of evaluation, and raises some crucial questions in the context of evaluating the 'merit' of health promotion initiatives and policies. For example, a reduction in the incidence of a disease over a specified period of time might be attributable to a particular intervention (such as the introduction of a clean water supply), a better take-up of vaccination or improved access to screening. These consequences are usually expressed in quantifiable sets of statistics, which might be used as a proxy measure of the effectiveness of a policy or practice. However, PIs more often measure neither effectiveness nor outcomes, but only outputs.

For example, Public Health Wales's (PHW) annual report for 2015–16 lists a number of comparative percentages for the past three years in the section 'Performance Analysis' (Public Health Wales, 2016b, Table 1, pp 37–38). These figures allow policy makers, practitioners and the public to see how the organisation has performed. But in what sense? The 'uptake of all scheduled childhood vaccinations at age 4' is less than the previous two years, as was the 'influenza vaccination uptake among the over-65s'. Exactly why there has been a relative reduction in both cases is not given (or perhaps not known). On the other hand, 'breast screening uptake' has shown an upturn in 'performance'. To what can this very welcome statistic be attributed?

Public Health England's (PHE) 2016 annual report adopts a similar PI approach in its summary of progress towards protecting and improving the public's health (Public Health England, 2016, pp 63–64). It lists a number of research-based activities in the fight against diseases abroad such as Ebola. One of the shortcomings of PIs is that the yardstick applied is primarily or exclusively input- and process-orientated. That means that those adopting this approach recount the resources (such as funding and staff) utilised for a particular intervention and the means by which those resources were applied. But even though the inputs and process might fulfil the objective of being 'of merit', other yardsticks – such as whether the *outputs, outcome* and *impact* matched the intended consequences – are not always reported. How these three components of an evaluation exercise may be defined will be dealt with later in this chapter.

But even if the outcomes and impact are proved to be successful, the questions 'what works?' and 'at what cost?' are not adequately answered. PHE (2016) accepts that this potential omission needs to be addressed, and includes a section in its report on health economics. (The role of health economics in health promotion is the subject of Chapter Five.) For example, the organisation has commissioned cost-effective prevention services for mental health and wellbeing and other cost-effective procedures (pp 27–30). In its analysis of performance over the preceding years, PHE follows the same pattern of data collection as its Wales counterpart.

This is not to be taken as an adverse criticism. PIs have their own value in the quest to discover whether health promotion 'works'. Carter et al. (1992) describe PIs as 'tin openers', because they can be used to clarify important questions about what they are actually telling us about performance as construed from different perspectives. This is the value of PIs at their best in the context of service evaluations: they can act as the starting point for closer and deeper analysis that is intended to provide answers to what might be called 'the so-what? question' (Palfrey et al., 2012).

Unfortunately, PIs can also be used to support a particular standpoint or ideological premise. This abuse is at its most malign when it purports to make comparisons between hospitals and schools. Much of this intended rivalry, initiated by governments, takes little or no account of variables that are likely to explain what would appear to be 'failing' organisations. This annual auditing stems from an insistence on devising targets that are meant to indicate the performance level at which different institutions are operating. In relation to hospitals, these include:

• waiting times for admission;
• waiting times for operations;

- ambulance response times;
- delayed transfer of care from hospital to the community.

Performance against these targets is also compared within the UK across its four nations.

A similar policy is implemented in education, in which Programme for International Student Assessment (PISA) scores are compared not only within the UK but also across other countries. PISA tests 15-year-old pupils in more than 70 countries in science, mathematics and reading. It must be assumed that these tests are standardised as far as possible across all the countries. At the last assessment, Singapore came top in all three subjects and the UK twenty-seventh. So, what does this tell us? What inferences can be drawn from these statistics, and what impact might they have on future education policies? Some countries have taken relatively poor results to justify changes to teacher training, but these and other resulting changes are not necessarily justified by what could be called 'crude data', as Rey (2010, p 17) argued: 'Such uses and interpretations often assume causal relationships that cannot legitimately be based upon PISA data which would normally require fuller investigation through qualitative in-depth studies and longitudinal surveys based on quantitative and qualitative methods'.

Rey's (2010) comment could equally apply to possibly unjustified inferences drawn from reported figures relating to hospital and ambulance waiting times. What are the ambulance response times in rural as opposed to urban areas, and if different target times have been set, how is each type of area defined? Comparing differences in waiting times for admission to hospitals, is it known whether different staffing levels across hospitals are taken into consideration, and are there divergences in the overall management of various wards? Without further probing analysis, the raw data remain a mere starting point for additional, non-quantitative enquiries. When discussing the usefulness and limitations of PIs, the definition of 'performance' requires clarification. In the case of the PHE and PHW annual reports, the issue is whether the planned *outputs* have been attained. This is important because the outputs are targeted as a means towards achieving the overriding objective of improving people's health and preventing illnesses.

Apart from PIs, two methods designed to generate hard data on the effectiveness and cost-effectiveness of health promotion policies and projects can contribute to gathering sound information. These are RCTs and interviews.

RCTs

Initial criticisms of RCTs did not prevent them becoming the 'gold standard' of research methods to test the effectiveness of medical interventions. This experimental research design relies on the willing participation of groups of people with similar characteristics, such as age, gender, socioeconomic circumstances and ethnicity. Participants are then assigned randomly to the experimental group or the control group. For example, in a clinical experiment to test a drug for its effectiveness in curing or delaying the onset of a disease, the subjects (and in some cases the experimenters) are 'blind', in that they do not know whether the group is accessing the drug or being given a placebo with no medical value. After a prescribed length of time, both groups are tested to discover whether the trial drug has proved effective.

It is possible to adapt the RCT approach in the context of a health promotion project. One example would be a 'quit smoking' programme in which individuals are matched for their smoking habits (such as numbers of cigarettes smoked per day) and for any other variable considered relevant to the project (such as age). A number of individuals would be assigned to the 'quit smoking' programme, while the others would remain outside this facility. After a certain length of time, both sets – the experimental group and the control group – would then be interviewed to find out whether the programme had had the desired effect. Merely recording the findings would not be enough; *why* there had or had not been a noticeable difference in the smoking habits of the experimental group would need to be explored. This second stage of the evaluation would seem obvious for reaching any conclusions about whether the project had been worthwhile. Yet critics such as Pawson and Tilley (1997) have argued that 'evaluators need to penetrate below the surface of observable inputs and outputs of a program' (p 216). They make what would seem to be a fairly obvious conclusion: that it is not sufficient to find out *whether* the hoped-for outcomes have been successfully achieved; it is imperative to know *how* and *for whom* they have (or have not) been achieved.

In the 'quit smoking' scenario, it would also be imperative to learn whether any reduction in smoking brought about by the project was sustained over a significant period, and whether there was any way to verify individuals' reporting of such changes. The answers to these two questions would be equally crucial in cases in which there had been no appreciable smoking reduction. In any experiment, whether in the laboratory or in the outside world, it can be extremely difficult to control all possible reasons why that experiment has failed or succeeded. For smokers to kick the habit, reduce their consumption or move to vaping, other factors might have played a part – such as an increase in the cost of cigarettes, encouragement and support from the family or a deterioration in health. Perhaps, in the field of health promotion, there might only rarely be cast-iron evidence that a particular intervention has achieved the ultimate objective of prevention or improvement. The danger lies in accepting the process and/or the output of a project as the end point of the evaluation.

A linear model of evaluation

Inputs → Process → Outputs → Outcomes → Impact

While it is not problematic to decide and assess the desired output of a health promotion project, formulating a proposed outcome might be difficult if this is also to be subject to an evaluation. To take an example from the PHE programme, the informing policy is 'to tackle child obesity'. At this point, it is necessary to clarify what is meant by *project, programme* and *policy*.

- **Project**: A planned activity aiming to achieving specified goals within a prescribed period.
- **Programme**: A set of separate planned activities unified into a coherent group.

- **Policy**: A statement of how an organisation or government would respond to particular eventualities or situations according to its values and principles. (Palfrey et al., 2012, p 33)

Van der Knaap (1995) confirmed these distinctive characteristics: 'policy evaluation is concerned with a thorough investigation into the implementation and effects of public policy (for example, a program, a project)' (p 200).

The essence of not only the child obesity project but also all of PHE's activities is to improve the public's 'health' and wellbeing. This broad objective is further dissected into *how* this will be achieved; that is, to secure the greatest gains in health and wellbeing and reductions in inequalities through evidence-based interventions. The main elements in PHE's policy to tackle child obesity are:

- a project to recruit 135,000 new parents into the Start4Life Information Service for Parents and 750,000 new registrations with Change4Life;
- supporting the development and implementation of a national childhood obesity strategy;
- supporting an increase in local physical activity by promoting tools, new initiatives and the latest evidence, particularly on sedentary behaviour and its impact.

It must therefore be assumed that either these three parts of the child obesity programme are already evidence-based or that their efficacy will be tested over the period that the programme is in operation.

It is important to go beyond assessing the output of a health promotion intervention and to evaluate the *outcome* – the result in terms of the stated objective. In the case of 'tackling' child obesity, this could be preventing a specific number or percentage of targeted children from becoming obese, or enabling the parent(s) to make sure that their child(ren) lose(s) weight. Most health promotion projects and programmes are likely to be longitudinal, in that it will take some time to allow the intervention to take effect. It is equally challenging to perceive the *impact* of the intervention on those participating. The distinction between *outcome* and *impact* can be illustrated in the case of a young person who has progressed from being obese to being of what might be termed 'normal weight'. There has been a successful outcome, but there might also have been a positive impact, in the sense of a strong effect or influence. Previously the child or young person might have been bullied about their size, but after the successful outcome this might no longer happen. This example also has a bearing on different dimensions of the concept of 'health'.

Adopting a linear model of health promotion evaluation reflects a tendency to visualise it as a clear, stage-by-stage progression. However, the input might have to be modified during the course of a project; for example, if funding is curtailed – or, indeed, increased. Similarly, the predesigned process of how the project will be implemented could prove unworkable or, after feedback from participants, might need to change to improve its chances of success. This could be described as *monitoring and surveillance*.

Two extended health promotion projects

Two schemes in Wales exemplify the benefits of long-term projects in enabling public health practitioners and policy makers to gain evidence for the effectiveness or otherwise of a particular project or programme.

The National Exercise Referral Scheme (NERS)

This is a 16-week programme including 'motivational interviewing, goal setting and relapse prevention' (Murphy et al., 2012, p 1). Twelve local health boards referred 2,160 inactive participants for risk of coronary heart disease; mild to moderate anxiety; or depression, stress or both. One group received the NERS; the other received normal care and brief written information. Outcome measures after 12 months included the seven-day physical activity recall and the hospital anxiety and depression scale. NERS was effective in increasing physical activity among those referred for coronary heart disease risk only. Among mental health referrals, NERS did not influence physical activity but was associated with reduced anxiety and depression. Effects were dependent on adherence, and it was found that NERS was likely to be cost-effective.

The authors selected NERS because:

> it is widely recognised that regular physical activity is beneficial to both physical and mental health. It is associated with reduced risk from chronic diseases, including chronic heart disease (CHD) and has been shown to be positively linked to mental health, including depression. Exercise referral schemes (ERS) can target specific patient or population subgroups with such conditions by providing contact with qualified exercise professionals (EP) and access to tailored programmes promoting physical activity. (Murphy et al., 2012, p 1)

The authors state that, despite the rapid growth of ERS in the UK, the evidence base for their effectiveness and cost-effectiveness is equivocal. In six previous RCTs, results were consistent with previous reviews of research trials; that is, there was a modest improvement in activity of individuals who were slightly active, but these increases were not maintained. Analysis after the termination of the scheme showed that effectiveness was highly dependent on adherence to the programme, with statistically significant differences in all outcomes among those who completed the 16-week programme compared with those who attended partially or not at all. For both mental health outcomes, the beneficial effect of the intervention was more apparent among women.

Overall, for patients referred for mental health reasons, the scheme did not increase their physical activity. It did, however, benefit them in terms of reduced anxiety and depression – particularly among women and younger patients. This suggested that the attention of the EP and the social contact and support generated by attendance may have been the reasons for improvements for these participants, rather than increased physical activity. It should be noted that, although clinicians referred patients who in their estimation were sedentary, several participants classified themselves as active or moderately active.

This NERS intervention was meticulously prepared according to the demands of an RCT research design, and called on rigorous statistical techniques to analyse the resulting data. It would be unwise to infer from this scheme that any increase in physical activity had improved the physical condition of the CHD patients. It did, however, indicate that tests on the anxiety and depression scales strongly suggested positive effects on the mental health cohort. In addition, increase in physical activity was greater in the experimental group than in the control group. With reference to the earlier section on outputs, outcomes and impact, this research confirmed a partial success in output (that is, increased physical activity) and, in the case of mental health participants, a successful outcome; that is, an improvement in their mental health. Analysis of the cost-effectiveness of the scheme will be mentioned in Chapter Five.

The Caerphilly Cohort Study

This research study was rather different from most other health promotion initiatives in that it did not involve an active project. It involved monitoring the health of 2,235 men aged 45–59 in the south Wales town of Caerphilly over a period of 30 years. The study began in 1980, and the results were recorded in a research paper in 2013 (Elwood et al., 2013). A large number of tests were carried out on the participants and questionnaires completed. Approximately every five years the men attended for re-examination; many of the tests were repeated and new ones added. The incentive to carry out the research was the fact that lifestyle and healthy behaviours are powerful determinants of morbidity and mortality (Reeves and Rafferty, 2005; Ford et al., 2011). The major concerns were smoking, body weight, physical exercise, alcohol consumption and diet. There is also some evidence that physical activity is associated with cognitive health (Sabia et al., 2009; Small et al., 2013), although the studies call for much longer-term research, since the processes linked to dementia and Alzheimer's disease are known to begin many years before detectable cognitive impairment (Sperling et al., 2011).

In their report, Elwood and colleagues summarised the evidence on the relationship between healthy lifestyles and the incidence of diabetes; vascular disease; cancer; all-cause mortality, cognitive impairment and dementia. Changes in adopting healthy behaviours were also monitored over the 30 years. The present or most recent occupation of each individual was used to derive social class, as in the Office of National Statistics classification, which was recorded as 'manual' or 'nonmanual'. After the baseline data was collected on behaviours related to the five lifestyle components, records were updated at five-year intervals when the men were re-questioned and re-examined and primary care and hospital records inspected to identify any new cases of type 2 diabetes, heart disease and possible stroke symptoms. Notifications of deaths and cancer registrations were also recorded. In the second re-examination of the men (aged 55–69) cognitive function was introduced into the study, and when the original cohort were aged 70–85 they were assessed for dementia.

At the start of the research study, 46% of the 2,235 men were nonsmokers and 35% had a healthy body mass index (BMI) of 18 to 24.9. Only 15% consumed five or more portions of fruit and/or vegetables daily. When this last statistic was reduced to three or more portions, 18% of participants satisfied this criterion. 'Regular exercise' was defined as about 30 minutes of light to moderate physical activity on at least five days each week; 39% said they took this, and 59% stated they drank within the guidelines of three or fewer units per day. At the outset of the study, 8% of men followed none of the healthy behaviours; 31% followed one behaviour; 36% followed two behaviours; 19% followed three, 5% followed four or five and just two men (0.1%) followed all five. The results of the study were as follows:

- The risk of *diabetes* declined as the number of healthy behaviours followed increased, as did the risk for *vascular disease*.
- *Cancer incidence* was not related to lifestyle, although there was a reduction in cancer associated with nonsmoking alone. There was also a reduction of one fifth in the number of *strokes* and *heart attacks*.
- There was a significant association between lifestyle and *all-cause mortality*.

- A detailed examination of results indicated that exercise is an important predictor of both *cognitive impairment* and *dementia*.
- The men who had a *healthy body weight* (BMI of 18 to 24.9) in 1980 experienced 20% fewer heart attacks and strokes than men with a higher BMI. In addition, almost 70% fewer men with low BMIs became diabetic over the 30 years.
- There did not appear to be any association between *alcohol intake* and health over the 30-year period.

Following a regime of more healthy behaviours was associated with reductions in several chronic diseases and mortality. There was a 50% reduction in diabetes, 50% in vascular diseases and 60% for all-cause mortality. The results after 30 years of research provide important data on the correlation between lifestyle and cognitive impairment and dementia, with a 60% reduction in both conditions. Overall, these results closely resemble the data produced by two studies in the US and another in Europe (Stampfer et al., 2000; Chiuve et al., 2006; Khaw et al., 2008). According to Elwood et al. (2013), the absence of any reduction in cancers other than by not smoking is surprising. Some research has shown reductions attributable to other healthy behaviours, but reduction in cancers appears to be highly variable and usually small (McCullough et al., 2011). In the Caerphilly study, the postponement of vascular disease for up to 12 years by healthy living and up to six years for death is interesting; these figures are based on the cases of all but two of the participants who followed four rather than all five healthy behaviours. In short, this 30-year study confirms that there is a substantial health benefit associated with a healthy lifestyle.

The location of the cohort study was selected because its social class distribution of the residents was considered to be (and remains) similar to that of the UK as a whole. The annual expenditure on prevention and public health services in Wales was estimated to be around £260 million, and the cost of unhealthy living to the NHS in Wales accounted for 10% of its total budget (Hale et al., 2012). Yet despite increasing public knowledge of the relevance of lifestyle to health and to survival, the proportion of the adult Welsh population adopting all five healthy behaviours remains under 1% (Elwood et al.,

2013). Elwood and his colleagues conclude their paper on the Caerphilly Cohort Study with this rather ominous warning:

Clearly there is an urgent need for new strategies in health promotion to be developed and evaluated. The costs of health services are increasing globally, and are likely to be unsustainable unless members of the public become more fully engaged and take a greater responsibility for their own health. Personal prevention measures, such as we describe, could have a large impact on the costs of healthcare services. Ultimately however, decisions about behaviours lie with the individuals and there is therefore an urgent need to establish a more effective partnership between health services and citizens. (Elwood et al., 2013, p 5)

These comments reflect a call for participation and empowerment in the development and application of health education and health promotion, which will be the subject of later sections in this chapter.

Alternatives to RCTs: qualitative methods

Potvin and Jones's (2011) statement that health promotion is process-orientated and needs to show outcomes raises the issue of which research methods other than RCTs are likely to generate valid and useful data – 'useful' in the sense of providing undisputed information about the ways in which health promotion has contributed to the health and wellbeing of individuals and, in some cases, communities. Elwood and his colleagues did not use RCTs, but applied the variable of 'number of health behaviours' to compare health outcomes over a lengthy period. They used validated tests to ascertain participants' health statuses (both physical and mental) as the research continued. They also used hospital data and questionnaires to gather baseline information and further information at five-yearly intervals. The participants were asked to inform the researchers about their current and later behaviours relating to smoking, physical activity, diet and alcohol consumption. Needless to say, here the evidence relied solely on the men giving truthful responses. For this reason, some of the more qualitative data collection methods could call into question the reliability of the data. A combination of qualitative and quantitative methods of assessing the performance of a health promotion initiative is often used.

Focus groups

As Thorogood and Coombes (2010) point out, focus groups can be involved in a health promotion project at all three stages: planning and design, implementation and evaluation. For example, they can be used when developing questions to be used in a questionnaire. In many cases, focus group participants will be the experts in a particular field. When exploring the reasons why some people appear to be averse to messages informing them about the risks of smoking and poor diet, people living in a socioeconomically deprived environment could advise public health practitioners of the key issues that need to be addressed. They might also offer help in how to devise jargon-free questions. In some studies, focus groups have been the sole means of gaining information, such as an evaluation of a quality-of-life questionnaire (Thorogood and Coombes, 2010).

As well as contributing to the planning and design stage of a health promotion initiative, a focus group could be vital in feeding back on the implementation stage of the project; for example, exploring why there has been very little uptake of the programme being implemented – or, conversely, why a programme is attracting a very high level of participation. The value of a participatory approach to the design and implementation stages of a health promotion project is linked to the concept of 'empowerment', which will be discussed later in this chapter. Indeed, Fetterman et al. (1995) refer to the involvement of individuals and communities as 'empowerment evaluation'. There may, however, be obstacles to overcome if the inclusion of laypersons in the project is not to become merely tokenistic. A paper published by Charities Evaluation Services (1998) sets out these potential difficulties:

- Involving users requires a lot of time and staff resources.
- Users may not want to be involved. Some may find the very idea of participation oppressive. Evaluators need to distinguish between a 'right' and a 'duty' to participate.
- Participatory approaches demand new roles for evaluators. Fully involving users of a service, project or programme means adopting the role of a facilitator rather than an expert.
- Involving people may raise expectations and lead to disappointment. Coote (1997) has warned that, if people are led to believe that their views will carry some weight with decision-makers and they then find that nothing happens as a result, they are likely to become cynical about the whole process.
- Involving individuals as research interviewers might lead policy makers to doubt the validity of the data produced.

Focus groups and individual interviews have the potential to make a valuable contribution to project or programme design, implementation and evaluation, but to make these the *only* sources of data might prove inadequate. On the other hand, their merit in discovering why some people persist in unhealthy behaviours would appear to be disregarded in too many health promotion initiatives.

Other qualitative methods

According to Thorogood and Britton (2010), RCTs are useful for measuring the *effects* of health promotion interventions, but not for explaining *why* these effects occur. To some exponents of RCTs, this might seem a rather contentious claim. RCTs' experimental design of having one group access an input (such as a quit smoking programme) but withholding it from the control group enables identification of whether it was the input that caused a reduction in smoking habits. As mentioned earlier, attempts must be made to exclude the possibility of extraneous factors influencing the outcome.

One way to do this is to arrange for further analysis of the results. The main qualitative methods that could produce additional information as to why a particular process or intervention did or did not have the intended effect are as follows.

Questionnaires

Positive: can provide a large number of anonymous responses and can be administered over a brief period.

Negative: some responses might be unclear, ambiguous and difficult to classify.

Personal interviews

Positive: may provide in-depth information and lend a new perspective on the health promotion initiative being evaluated.

Negative: often time-consuming and might not be free from interviewer bias.

Observation

Positive: capable of interpreting attitudes towards certain aspects of a project or programme.

Negative: Participants' awareness of being observed could affect their behaviour.

These and other methods listed by Aceijas (2011), such as checklists, case studies and minutes of meetings, may play an important part in offsetting the possibility of gathering partial or inaccurate information.

Two other methods of implementing a health promotion intervention are available if a randomised controlled test is considered either unfeasible or inappropriate. One is the **quasi-experimental design.** Instead of individuals being assigned on a random basis to the experimental or control group, a comparison group is selected in which the participants are similar to the experimental group in important characteristics such as age, gender or ethnicity. The other method could be a **before-and-after study.** In this case, a pre-test is followed by the intervention and a post-test is then applied. This was the core method used in the Caerphilly Cohort Study.

Health promotion towards 'empowerment'

Chapter One introduced the term 'empowerment' as a key aim of health promotion. The objective of health promotion policies, programmes and projects to empower individuals and communities deserves consideration, not least because it needs to be clearly defined. Green and Tones (2012) stress the need for empowerment, but what this means in practical terms remains unclear. The World Health Organization (WHO) refers to health promotion as a process of enabling people to increase control over, and to improve. their health (WHO, 1984). This policy statement refers to individual and community empowerment. Laverack (2009) points out that 'whereas health education is aimed at informing people to influence their individual or collective decision-making, health promotion aims at complementary social and political actions, such as advocacy and community development' (p 10). He criticises top-down approaches to improving people's health, in which the 'experts' 'pre-define the objectives, strategic approach, means of implementation, budget and time frame' (p 64).

Laverack (2009) also points out the contradiction in many programmes that have 'citizen empowerment' as a key objective but a 'top-down' approach to design, monitoring and evaluation. Top-down approaches can be disempowering, especially to those who are socially disadvantaged – who, ironically, are the intended beneficiaries of the programme. Such an approach can reinforce people's feelings of powerlessness by ignoring their concerns, overriding their needs and giving the message that their problems are not relevant to those who hold power – notably, the health promotion 'experts'. Top-down interventions run the risk of coercing the community into being involved with issues that are not a priority to them but that they are expected to participate in and contribute towards. Laverack (2009) concludes by spelling out the three essential elements of a truly collaborative engagement between health promotion initiators and the public:

- respect for all parties as equal yet possessing different values, concerns and meanings, all of which are equally important;
- a determination to seek all parties' perceptions;

- an opportunity for all to discuss and interpret the findings in order to reach a consensus on the best explanation. (Laverack, 2009, p 118)

Tones (2001) makes a similar criticism of the top-down approach, which he associates with the inappropriate application of RCTs as the primary research design. He dismisses RCTs in the pursuit of health promotion initiatives on a number of grounds:

- They are difficult to achieve in practice.
- Random allocation is difficult and artificial.
- There are often ethical issues in withholding health promotion from individuals and communities.
- Contamination is almost inevitable when trying to compare experimental areas with control or comparison areas in large-scale interventions.
- Health promotion usually involves a complex multifactorial intervention; it is dramatically different from the provision of medication, for which the RCT might well be suitable.
- As Thorogood and Britton (2010) commented, RCTs might indicate that a given intervention has been successful or not, but we would not normally know why.

Community empowerment

In contrast with a top-down approach to designing, implementing and evaluating a health promotion initiative, there has been a discernible campaign to engage with communities, enabling them to take a much more assertive role in decisions about healthcare services and how to improve health. In England, the Local Government and Public Involvement in Health Act 2007 required public bodies, including health trusts and hospital foundations, to work with their local communities in ways that give them a greater say over decisions. The Act came into force in 2009. A year earlier, the Department of Health (2008) published the document *Taking the lead: Engaging people and communities.* However, Gregson and Court (2010) reduced the term 'engagement' to a second-level policy in their report on building health communities. The Act of 2007 did stress that engagement went beyond merely 'consulting'. In their report, Gregson and Court (2010) emphasised the need to empower communities so as to bring about improvement in health. This report does not specifically define the concept of 'community'.

The Calouste Gulbenkian Foundation (1984), however, described 'community' as a grouping of people who share a common purpose, interest or need and who can express their relationship through face-to-face communication, as well as other means, without difficulty and usually in the same locality. Laverack and Wallerstein (2001) also refer to common interests and needs, but add that a community is able to mobilise and organise itself towards social and political change. The salient phrase here is 'organise itself'. This suggests people *taking* power, not being *given* it by those who have the real power to bring about change. Gregson and Court, writing under the aegis of the Community Development Foundation, perceive empowerment not as a means of gaining greater influence over external conditions normally beyond people's influence or control, but rather as enabling people to become more aware of how they can take responsibility for maintaining their own health. They regard this as particularly important for 'people from disadvantaged communities facing greater levels of risk from smoking, alcohol misuse, accidents and poor diet' (p 25). They add: 'Community members are often well aware of the underlying causes of poor health because they understand the conditions that create or perpetuate illness. By helping communities to investigate and articulate these, healthcare providers can devise remedies that suit local circumstances and tackle the real issues in people's lives' (p 25).

As will be evident in Chapter Four, many commentators would challenge the claim that healthcare providers themselves have the power to remedy circumstances that are outside the remit of healthcare organisations. They would espouse a much more radical approach to changing what they would regard as the root cause of health inequalities: poverty, substandard housing and unemployment. The report on behalf of the Community Development Foundation in England is keen to delineate the advantages to be gained from working with communities to help them exert more influence over health policies and projects. It provides a summary of ten initiatives in various parts of England. All these schemes reflect the commitment and energy that has gone into engaging with local residents, both adults and children. There have been training courses to produce community 'champions' and, in general, the results of all ten schemes have been hailed as successful. Yet no evidence is presented of the projects achieving the core objective that informs all community empowerment interventions; that is, creating 'healthier communities'. As in so many reports of health promotion activities, the 'success' lies in the outputs that have been produced; that is, individuals being more informed about how to improve their health. This implies that, in today's world, changing people's lifestyles is the key to bringing about health improvements and reducing health inequalities – not building social and political pressure to change the financial, social and environmental conditions over which ordinary people have no control.

In Scotland, the Community Empowerment Scotland Act 2015 visualises the special contribution that empowered communities can make towards creating a more prosperous and fairer Scotland. Where communities are empowered, the Scottish Government would expect to see a range of benefits, such as increased confidence and skills among local people, higher numbers of people volunteering, better quality of life and people in the same locality having more opportunity to buy land and buildings. Recently, Durham University set up a research project to compare progress in England and Scotland under the title *Reframing citizen relationships with the public sector in a time of austerity*, which focuses in particular on how community empowerment is changing in both countries (Painter and Pande, 2013).

Results

There is considerable agreement within the UK that health promotion has a duty to enable people to have more power over their health development. A current term that encapsulates an increased partnership between health professionals and lay people is **coproduction**. This is a long way from the notion of a patient in the original sense of that word as someone who bears or suffers. Coproduction establishes a new relationship between someone who seeks medical help and one who provides it. This asserts that both patient and medic are experts who need each other's assistance in deciding the most appropriate and beneficial response to a perceived health issue. This might lead to a particular treatment or to watchful waiting. It is essentially a form of citizen empowerment.

Naturally, there is no obligation on the part of the person seeking assistance or advice to accept the professional's advice. In the context of health promotion, those individuals who do not heed or act upon information about the health hazards of leading what the professional would consider an unhealthy lifestyle possess the ultimate power to ignore the advice. Health promotion specialists do not grant them that power; it is enshrined in law that in matters of health, apart from exceptional circumstances, each citizen has the right to make their own decisions. The exponents of what might be termed a **socioecological** view of what can determine whether a person is able to follow a healthy lifestyle would, however, contend that this 'right' is seriously undermined by poor living conditions and low income.

A major problem in the quest for community empowerment is how to measure the outcomes of relevant schemes and exercises. Davies and Macdonald (1998) addressed this question, noting that many health promotion interventions relied on short-term outcomes relating to increased knowledge and attitude. They also argued that: 'It is crucially important ... to clarify whose objectives are being pursued when carrying out assessment of quality and effectiveness' (p 207). In evaluating whether citizen and community empowerment has been achieved, we need to know not only the formal evaluators' interpretation of a 'before-and-after' scenario but also whether those targeted to be empowered consider their situation to have changed for the better in terms of decision-making – but also, and more importantly, in terms of their current and previous state of health.

Empowerment evaluation

In the 1970s and 1980s, Guba and Lincoln introduced the idea of collaborative evaluation. In this process, the evaluator collaborates with programme stakeholders through all stages in the evaluation process. Stakeholders – the subjects of the project – are not viewed solely as sources of data but are seen as having an important part to play in deciding the nature, form and content of the evaluation. They labelled this evaluation paradigm **fourth-generation evaluation** (Guba and Lincoln, 1989). This concept was further developed by Fetterman (1994), who described the key elements and purpose of empowerment evaluation: 'Empowerment evaluation is the use of evaluation to help others help themselves. It is designed to foster self-determination, rather than dependency. Empowerment evaluation focuses on improvement, is collaborative, and requires both qualitative and quantitative methodologies' (p 305). Fetterman regards this revised role of the evaluator as a moral duty, especially when a health-orientated piece of research is directed towards people who are marginalised, economically disadvantaged and powerless. They are then enabled to 'shape the direction of the evaluation, suggest ideal solutions to their problems, and then take an active role in making social change happen' (Fetterman, 1994, p 6). Empowerment evaluation, according to Fetterman, can be a liberating experience for individuals, groups, organisations and communities (Clarke, 1999).

Nevertheless, there can be an inherent complication in collaborative or empowerment evaluation. This could happen when stakeholders are granted a say in the actual evaluation but some groups within the 'community' may find that they are given little, if any, opportunity to influence the programme itself: 'Viewed cynically, this possible effect of stakeholder-based evaluation could be seen as a means of social control, rather than empowerment, by which the powerful appease the less powerful by giving the appearance of control without relinquishing any power' (Mark and Shotland, 1985). This viewpoint would seem to have particular relevance in health promotion projects in which the explicit objective is to confront and reduce, if not eradicate, health inequalities. Fetterman's (1994) aforementioned point about 'making social change happen' must be an extremely challenging aim for both external evaluator and intended beneficiaries of the health promotion activity. If, as the next chapter will indicate, many commentators are correct in arguing that attempts to prevent illness and disease by trying to help people adopt a healthier lifestyle are entirely misplaced, then social change will never happen. Empowerment evaluation can certainly be valued as an attempt to accord a more influential role in the design, process and assessment of the project or programme, but many argue that this alone will not lead to the necessary social change.

Concluding thoughts

When discussing formal evaluation, it is perhaps wise to neither portray it as some esoteric exercise nor to state the obvious. Hubley and Copeman (2008) manage to avoid both these extremes, instead offering some clear guidelines and presenting a list of possible impediments to achieving meaningful and valid data on which to base future action. The technical terms – **internal** and **external validity** – are explained in this way:

> A health promotion intervention might have been successful in one context, but the same success might not be achieved in another, where the local community may have a different culture/ethnic background. ... When looking at an evaluation report of a health promotion intervention you need to consider whether there were any special features in that community that contributed to its success and, if so, whether the same success could be achieved if the approach was repeated elsewhere. (Hubley and Copeman, 2008, p 343)

They then list some possible problems in drawing conclusions about the effectiveness of the intervention:

- No objectives/targets were set at the beginning, so the purpose of the programme was not clear.
- The objectives/targets are not measurable because they were set out in terms that were too general (for example, 'increase exercise', 'increase awareness', 'empower people').
- No baseline study was carried out, so it is not possible to demonstrate any improvement as a result of the health promotion activity.
- Unanticipated benefits or negative outcomes are not picked up.
- The evaluation was focused on the achievement or nonachievement of the objectives, so other changes were not noticed.
- A lack of impact is demonstrated, but reasons for failure are not known because insufficient supporting information was collected.
- An impact is demonstrated, but it could be for reasons other than the programme. A lack of controls or supporting information make it difficult to prove that the change was a result of the health promotion.
- The benefits of the health promotion are seen only after the end of the programme and are not noticed in the evaluation.
- Improvements in the community are not sustained and the situation reverts back to the original state. (Hubley and Copeman, 2008, p 344)

They conclude with some advice that features prominently in the work of Palfrey et al. (2012) on 'evaluation for the real world':

> In reviewing evaluations, you need to recognize that in the real world nothing is ever perfect. Evaluation is not easy and most assessments have flaws of some kind. You should take a positive approach and not dismiss an evaluation out of hand just because it contains some weaknesses. The challenge is to understand the limitations of an evaluation, learn what you can from it, but take care not to draw conclusions that are not supported by the findings. (Hubley and Copeman, 2008, p 344)

The point that Palfrey et al. (2012) make is that even though the evaluation may have concluded with an unequivocal set of data indicating that a particular intervention needs to be replicated in one context or another, those who have the authority to make decisions might, for any one of a number of reasons, decline to take any action. This issue will be discussed in Chapter Eight.

FOUR

Strategies for health promotion

Alternative interpretations of the route to better health

The following two opposing routes to better health could be described as **the two health promotion doctrines**. Approach A is a health education approach that seeks to influence individual lifestyle, while Approach B proposes social change and political action as the only way to reduce health inequalities and improve public health.

Approach A

- Don't smoke. If you can, stop. If you can't, cut down.
- Follow a balanced diet, with plenty of fruit and vegetables.
- Keep physically active.
- Manage stress by, for example, talking things through and making time to relax.
- If you drink alcohol, do so in moderation.
- Cover up in the sun and protect children from sunburn.
- Practise safer sex.
- Take up cancer-screening opportunities.
- Be safe on the roads: follow the Highway Code.
- Learn the First Aid ABC – airways, breathing, circulation.

Approach B

- Don't be poor. If you can, stop. If you can't, try not to be poor too long.
- Don't have poor parents.
- Own a car.
- Don't work in a stressful, low-paid, manual job.
- Don't live in damp, low-quality housing.
- Be able to go on a foreign holiday and sunbathe.
- Practise not losing your job and don't become unemployed.

- Take up all the benefits you are entitled to if you are unemployed, retired, sick or disabled.
- Don't live next to a busy major road or near a polluting factory.
- Learn how to fill in the complicated housing benefit/asylum application forms before you become homeless and destitute. (Raphael, 2002)

While epidemics of contagious diseases have disappeared from the UK, other health concerns have prompted all parts of the UK to declare policies to confront four quasi-epidemics: obesity, lack of exercise, poor diet and dementia. Just as in previous centuries, when faced with an epidemic, government health policies have focused on trying to establish the cause of what might be termed **serious health variations**. In the UK, all four governmental bodies have pinpointed socioeconomic factors as the most likely reasons why certain sections of the population are experiencing relatively poor health.

Causes of ill health

The question of whether poverty, however defined, is a cause of ill health has been discussed in previous chapters. What follows is a more detailed investigation into whether this is merely a supposition or whether it stems from undeniable research-based evidence. In addition, authoritative surveys and reports on health from the four constituent countries within the UK will be presented, including references to the prevalence of poverty in 21st-century Britain. A focus on child poverty will also feature in this chapter.

According to the Scottish Government's (2017) document *Bridging the gap: Poverty and health inequalities*, health inequalities are the result of a variety of interrelating factors, but a primary cause is poverty. In this document, people live in poverty 'when they are denied an income sufficient for their material needs and when these circumstances exclude them from taking part in activities which are an accepted part of daily life in that society' (p 1). This situation limits access to adequate housing and education as well as to essentials such as food, fuel and clothing. Socioeconomic disadvantage can lead to feelings of hopelessness and despair, which in turn can result in social exclusion. In addition, low birth weight, which has a strong association with deprivation, results in poorer health in adulthood. The children of low-income families are likely to have low levels of literacy and numeracy, while a low level of health literacy impacts on the ability to access appropriate services – including preventative health programmes – which results in poorer health outcomes. All these adverse circumstances are likely to lead to stress through a feeling of powerlessness: an inability to exercise some control over and manage one's health and life generally.

The Scottish Government's earlier document, *Equally well review* (2010a, p 2), made it clear that relatively poor health could not be attributed exclusively to an unhealthy lifestyle: 'Poor health is not simply due to diet, smoking or other lifestyle choices. We need to understand factors underlying poor health and health inequalities such as people's aspirations, sense of control and cultural factors.' Neither of the two documents proposes a course of action to tackle the problem of poverty and poor health.

Poverty in the UK

A Joseph Rowntree Foundation report (Tinson et al., 2016) takes up the same theme of poverty and social exclusion, and lists some statistics that detail a 'comprehensive picture of poverty in the UK' (p 2):

- In 2014–15, there were 13.5 million people living in low-income households – 21% of the UK population. This proportion has barely changed since 2002–03.
- The number of private renters in poverty has doubled over the past decade. Rent accounts for at least one third of income for more than 70% of private renters in poverty.
- The number of households accepted as homeless and the number of households in temporary accommodation have both increased for five years in a row. Evictions by landlords are near a ten-year high.
- The proportion of working-age adults in employment is at a record high. Full-time employees account for 62% of the

growth in jobs since 2010. The proportion of young adults who are unemployed is the lowest since 2005. However, the rising cost of living and the freeze on benefits and tax credits mean ordinary working families are struggling.

- The number of people in working families living in poverty is a record high of 55%. Four fifths of the adults in these families are themselves working, some 3.8 million workers. Those adults who are not working are predominantly looking after children.
- The number of children in long-term workless households is 1.4 million; down 280,000 in four years. Excluding lone-parent families with a child under five, 55% of these children have a disabled adult in their household. Four million children are living in poverty; this figure is expected to rise by 2021.

Trends in the incidence of poverty in the UK are not altogether bleak. As well as the increase in full-time employment, 400,000 fewer pensioners were in poverty, despite there being 1.7 million people aged 65 and over in the UK. The report is presented as 'a valuable resource for researchers and policy makers … it aims to better illuminate the challenges of tackling poverty' (Tinson et al., 2016, p 12). It offers guidance on some of the key challenges to be tackled. It argues that, in what it perceives to be a period of sustained economic growth, 'it is important that those on low incomes share in it and feel the gains' (p 11). Two relevant policy issues here are zero-hours contracts (Pyper and Dar, 2015) and the minimum wage, which was raised to £7.50 per hour in 2017 (up from £7.20). Tinson et al. (2016) do not attempt to draw conclusions about any correlation between poverty and health. Instead, they highlight some opportunities for *preventing* – not just *reducing* – the prevalence of poverty in the UK:

> But we must also consider how the economy and the state can be restructured to prevent poverty in the first place. Great progress has been made in reducing pensioner poverty, but progress on child poverty is at risk. Housing in the UK is too often expensive and of poor quality, particularly in the private rented sector. Work, although the best defence against low income,

is too often insufficient. The social security system has become less effective for those with housing costs and Council Tax to pay. (Tinson et al., 2016, p 11)

Defining poverty in the 20th and 21st centuries

If poverty is regarded as a key influence in adversely affecting the health of millions of people in the UK, there needs to be a universally accepted definition of the term. The yardstick applied by the UK government of less than 60% of the median household income as the definition of poverty has been challenged. Before this current definition was officially adopted, Peter Townsend (1979) proposed certain criteria that should be seriously considered. He preferred the term 'relative deprivation':

> Poverty can be defined objectively and applied consistently only in terms of the concept of relative deprivation. ... Individuals, families and groups in the population can be said to be in poverty when they lack the resources to obtain the types of diet, participate in the activities and have the living conditions and amenities which are customary, or at least widely encouraged or approved, in the societies to which they belong. (Townsend, 1979, p 1)

Townsend was not the first to use the term **relative deprivation** as preferable to the concept of **absolute poverty**; Stouffer coined the phrase in the US 30 years earlier (Stouffer et al, 1949), and Merton (1957) and Runciman (1966) later used it in their work on social structure and on social justice respectively. Seebohm Rowntree's survey in York (Rowntree, 1901) described families whose total earnings were insufficient to obtain the minimum necessaries for maintaining merely physical efficiency as being in **primary poverty**. Rowntree calculated the cost of food, clothing and fuel at a basic level to sustain a family and added rental costs. Townsend found this calculation too absolute and objective to serve as a precise depiction of poverty. He maintained that Rowntree's estimates of the costs of necessities other than food were based either on his own and others' opinions or, as in the case of clothing, on the actual expenditure of those among a small sample of poor families who spent the least.

In the case of food, estimates of the nutrients required were very broad averages and were not varied by age and family composition. The foods chosen to meet these estimates were selected arbitrarily, 'with a view to securing minimally adequate nutrition at lowest cost, rather than in correspondence with diets that are conventional among the poorer working classes' (Townsend, 1979, p 4). In addition, according to Townsend, people's needs – even for food – are conditioned by the society in which they live, and differ in different periods of the evolution of societies. For this reason, absolute definitions of poverty are misleading and unhelpful. Perhaps Townsend's most telling (and possibly provocative) assertion is that classifying some sections of the population as living in poverty is a value judgement. It is not something one can verify or demonstrate, except by inference and suggestion. However, in what could be interpreted as a contradictory statement, he adds that this does not mean that a definition cannot be objective and that it cannot be distinguished from social or individual opinion.

Townsend does not discuss any link between poverty – or relative deprivation – and health. This, however, is the main theme in Main and Bradshaw's (2016) book. They urge a move towards **redistributive policies**, which are rooted in the idea that structures within society unfairly disadvantage some people. By way of contrast, they argue that current policies in the UK arise from the belief that poverty is the result of poor individual choices and behaviours. These may be transmitted from one generation to the next, resulting in 'cultures of poverty'. As a result, action to address child poverty shifts from providing additional resources to poor families to helping poor parents to overcome personal shortcomings. Any increases in the percentage of the population in employment conceal the fact that the working poor are at the mercy of low pay, zero-hour contracts and downward social mobility.

Main and Bradshaw's (2016) survey found that adults living in poor households were likely to sacrifice their own needs to provide for their children. Many parents reported that they had:

- skimped on food so others would have enough to eat;
- bought second-hand clothes instead of new;
- continued to wear worn-out clothes;
- cut back on visits to the hairdresser or barber;
- postponed visits to the dentist;
- spent less on hobbies;
- cut back on social visits, going to the pub or eating out.

Lansley and Mack (2015) support their critique of the dominant governmental approach; that is, health promotion interventions focusing on improving health literacy and encouraging people to follow a healthier lifestyle.

Child poverty

In 2010, the UK government set a target of eradicating child poverty by 2020 (Child Poverty Act 2010). This target will not be achieved in any part of the UK. The health impact of children living in households below 60% of median income has been well-documented by organisations such as Barnardo's and the Child Poverty Action Group. Throughout the UK, poverty affects one in four children; that is, a person under the age of 18. This figure has risen to 2.3 million and is calculated to reach 3.6 million by 2020 (Child Poverty Action Group, 2016). Poverty, as currently defined, is not exclusively the result of adult unemployment. Two thirds of children growing up in poverty live in households in which at least one member of the family is working. Of those living in poverty, 34% are in families with three or more children. Because of this upward trend, a private members' bill – the Child Poverty in the UK (Target for Reduction) Bill 2016–17 – was due to have its second reading in parliament in May 2017. However, parliament was dissolved on 3 May 2017 because of the impending general election, so the Bill fell and no further action is to be taken.

In Northern Ireland, 101,000 children (24%) are deemed to be living in poverty (Barnardo's, 2016); but in Wales, one third of the child population lives in poverty, with 14% in severe poverty (a family at or below 50% of the median household income) (Save the Children, 2012). Recent analysis by the Joseph Rowntree

Foundation found that although employment was at record levels in 2017, nearly half of single-parent children were poor, with a particularly sharp rise among children of lone parents who work full time. About two thirds of the UK's poor children are from working families.

In Scotland, the Child Poverty Action Group not only reports on the proportion of children in poverty (1 in 4) but also the effects on health and action required to reduce this proportion. It defines 'children in poverty' as those growing up in families without the resources to obtain the type of diet, participate in the activities and have the living conditions and amenities that are the norm in 21st-century Scotland. The report cites the example of a two-parent family with two children aged 5 and 14 living on less than £401 per week, after housing costs have been deducted. In terms of health outcomes, three-year-olds in households with incomes below £10,000 per annum are two and a half times more likely to suffer chronic illness than children in households with incomes above £52,000 per annum. The report also states that there are strong links between the experience of child poverty and poor mental health. There is evidence that children living in low-income households are nearly three times as likely to suffer mental health problems as their more affluent peers.

The Child Poverty Action Group Scotland sets out five courses of action that it believes would ease the problem of poverty. These might well be applicable in the rest of the UK.

1 *Access to secure employment and decent pay*. Given that low pay and job insecurity are key factors in the existence of in-work poverty, it is essential that all working parents receive at least the living wage, a reasonable degree of security and opportunities to develop their skills and progress at work.
2 *Adequate social security benefits*. Benefit rates should be increased to a level that ensures children do not experience poverty, whether their parents are in or out of work.
3 *Increased uptake of benefits*. According to Department of Work and Pensions figures, between 19% and 23% of families in the UK are not claiming the means-tested benefits to which they are entitled. This highlights the need for more information and advice.

4 *Affordable childcare.* Overall, the average cost of part-time (25 hours) childcare in Scotland under two is £5,514 a year. As well as easing pressure on family budgets, increased provision of affordable childcare would facilitate access to employment for parents and carers.

5 *The removal of financial barriers to education.* The provision of free school meals could save a family with two children more than £800 a year. Providing adequate school clothing grants to low-income families and reducing the cost of school transport and school trips would also help to ease the financial pressure experienced by families.

Exceptions

Although there is convincing evidence that children in lower-income families are more likely than others to suffer relatively poor health, this is not universally true. For example, some of the poorest parts of England are bucking the trend that suggests that children's health is determined by where they live. The National Children's Bureau (NCB) (2015) analysed how many under-5s in each local authority were obese, had tooth decay, had been in hospital or were judged to be less emotionally, intellectually and physically developed. Deprivation was not uniformly linked to ill health; the report showed that poor early childhood outcomes are not inevitable for children growing up in deprived local authority areas (Moody, 2015). For example, among the 30 most deprived areas:

- Seven have average levels of obesity.
- One is in the best fifth for tooth decay, and another is in the second-best fifth.
- Another seven are in the best fifth for injury, and four are in the second-best fifth.
- Three are in the best fifth for showing a good level of development, and two are in the second-best fifth.

Furthermore, there is a noticeable variation in health status between areas that have similar levels of deprivation. The report recommends that Public Health England (PHE) and the

Department of Health conduct research to determine what local approaches are making a difference to children's health outcomes.

Health surveys

All constituent parts of the UK – England, Scotland, Wales and Northern Ireland – publish health surveys that provide an annual update on current health behaviours and conditions. These reports do not set out to explain the causes of these behaviours and conditions. They list certain information that tacitly relates lifestyle choices to illnesses, based on accepted epidemiological and clinical research.

England

Health Survey for England (2016)

The summary of key facts in this survey provides an annual monitoring of trends in the nation's health. This includes estimating the proportion of people who have specified health conditions and the prevalence of risk factors and behaviours associated with these conditions:

- *Adult smoking*: 19% of men and 17% of women were current smokers; 40% of smokers had tried e-cigarettes.
- *Adult alcohol consumption*: 31% of men and 16% of women drank over 14 units in a usual week.
- *Adult obesity*: 27% of adults were obese; 41% of men and 31% of women were overweight.
- *Children's physical activity*: Excluding school-based activities, 22% of children aged 5–15 met the physical activity guidelines of being at least moderately active for at least 60 minutes every day.
- *Children's smoking*: 1% of children aged 8–15 smoked at least one cigarette each week.
- *Children's drinking*: 1% of children aged 8–15 reported usually drinking once a week or more.

PHE (2016) Annual Report

One disturbing trend from previous years was the 18.6% increase in deaths from dementia and Alzheimer's disease. Two other causes for concern were the number of households living in temporary accommodation and a decrease in those presenting for breast and cervical screening. One positive statistic was that, compared with 2012–13, there were fewer children living in low-income households. The top five risk factors were listed as:

1 dietary risks
2 tobacco smoke
3 high body mass index
4 high systolic blood pressure
5 alcohol and drug misuse

And the main killer diseases:

1 heart disease
2 stroke
3 cancers
4 liver disease
5 lung disease

Townsend (2014) reported that men in the most deprived areas of England died on average at 74 years old, while those in the top tenth economically died on average at the age of 83. For women, the figures were 79 and 86 respectively. High rates of smoking and obesity contributed significantly to these disparities in mortality rates. In the same year, according to the Health and Social Care Information Centre (2016), 65% of men and 58% of women were obese; the highest levels were in the northeast of the country at 31% (compared with 21% in London). As a contrast, the same report shows that adult obesity levels in Japan were less than 5%.

For both adult and child obesity, the rates in deprived areas were double those in the more affluent regions. With regard to physical activity in adults, 57% reported no activity during the previous 28 days, and 41% of men compared with 31% of women played sport at least once a week.

Scotland

Scotland Health Survey 2016

The survey reported the following results for key risk factors and behaviours associated with adverse health conditions.

- Alcohol:
  - Those drinking above the recommended limit fell from 34% in 2003 to 26% in 2015.
  - Men drank twice as much as women.
  - Individuals drinking more than 14 units a week were more commonly found in the higher income groups (46%) than the lowest (11%).
  - Drinking levels generally declined with age.

- Smoking:
  - The percentage of people smoking decreased from 28% in 2003 to 21% in 2015.
  - Males smoked on average 13.9 cigarettes a day; females, 11.3.

- Diet:
  - Of adults, 21% reached the five-a-day fruit and vegetable target, and only 12% of children did so.
  - Consumption of the fruit and vegetable target was lowest in the 18–24 age group and highest among those aged 55–75.

- Physical activity:
  - 63% of adults met the recommended guidelines (67% of men; 59% of women).
  - 73% of children met the guidelines (77% of boys; 69% of girls).

- Obesity:
  - 65% of adults were overweight, of whom 29% were obese. This figure had hardly changed since 2005.
  - 15% of boys and 14% of girls were considered to be 'at risk' of obesity – the same percentage as in 1998.

Wales

The Annual Welsh Health Survey 2016

The following figures relate to the results of the 2015 survey.

- Alcohol:
  - 46% of men drank more than the guidelines for alcohol units compared with 33% of women. This statistic referred to intake on the previous day.
  - 15% of the sample were non-drinkers.
  - Consumption decreased as deprivation increased.

- Smoking:
  - 19% of adults smoked: 21% men; 18% women.
  - Adults in more deprived areas were the most likely to smoke.
  - The age at which adults smoked peaked between 25–34 years old.
  - 29% had given up smoking and 52% had never smoked.
  - 6% currently smoked e-cigarettes only. It was very rare for people who had never smoked to take up smoking e-cigarettes.

- Diet:
  - 32% ate at least five fruits and vegetables on the previous day. This represented a decline since 2008.
  - 64% of children ate fruit every day and 52% ate vegetables daily.

- Physical activity:
  - 58% reported undertaking at least 150 minutes of 'moderate physical activity' or 75 minutes of 'vigorous activity' each week.
  - 30% were inactive.
  - Physical activity decreased in the lower levels of deprivation.
  - 36% of children were physically active for at least an hour every day.

- Obesity:
  - 36% were overweight and 24% were obese.
  - Those in the 45–64 age range were most likely to be overweight or obese.
  - 63% of all adults in the most deprived areas were obese and 54% in the least deprived areas

Northern Ireland

Health Survey (NI): first results

As well as providing details relating to healthy (or unhealthy) diet and lifestyle, the Northern Ireland survey (Scarlett and Denvir, 2016) asked a sample of respondents about their decisions on what they ate, and asked them about what the Scottish Government's (2017) *Bridging the gap* referred to as 'health literacy'. These are the statistics.

- Alcohol:
  - 32% of men and 11% of women drank more than the official weekly limits.
  - This was a decrease from 37% of men and 15% of women five years ago.

- Smoking:
  - 25% of males and 20% of females smoked (a slight reduction over the past five years).

- Diet:
  - 37% ate five portions of fruit and vegetables each day (up from 33% in 2010–11).

- Obesity:
  - 65% of males and 57% of females were obese (classified as having a body mass index (BMI) of 30–39.9) or overweight (classified as having a BMI of 25–29.9).
  - 9% of children were obese and 16% were overweight.

Since 2011–12, the proportion of people eating fruit and vegetables on most days of the week had increased. However, there was an increase in the proportion of people eating processed meat, biscuits, sweets and chocolate. This is important information, since many surveys are likely to pose the question about fruit and vegetable intake without also asking about types of food considered less healthy. Comparisons were also made between food consumed by persons classified as 'most deprived' and those 'least deprived'; 68% of the most deprived ate fruit while 80% of the least deprived did so. There was also a difference of 13% with regard to consumption of vegetables between the two classifications. The most deprived also ate significantly more chips, processed meat and sweets and drank far more sugary or fizzy drinks than the least deprived. Without actually offering a definition of what the survey authors termed 'deprivation', the measure of that term was a combination of seven **deprivation domains**:

- income (this made up 25% of the total measure)
- employment (25%)
- health or disability (15%)
- education, skills and training (15%)
- proximity to services (10%)
- living environment (5%)
- prevalence of crime and disorder (5%)

One critical response from the 3,915 survey participants centred on the effect of low income on eating habits. Four percent of households indicated that on at least one day in the last fortnight they had not had a substantial meal due to lack of money, 2% said they sometimes did not have enough to eat and just under 1% said they often did not have enough to eat. In addition, while 85% always had enough of the kinds of food they wanted to eat, 13% had enough to eat but not always the kinds of food they wanted. Unfortunately, these last two percentages give no indication of the types of food the respondents wanted to eat. To have enough or not enough so-called 'junk food' to eat tells us nothing about financial capacity to buy the ingredients for a healthy meal. Statistics related to eating habits showed that 4% fewer people in the most deprived category than the least deprived category understood media information on how to improve their health. This might suggest that low-income people accept that their eating habits go against health promotion and health education campaigns to improve health and prevent illness.

Comment

The categories under which the health surveys gather data form the basis of most current health promotion policies and interventions, namely smoking, alcohol consumption, diet, physical activity and BMI. The surveys present the data, but do not attempt to analyse the causes of upward or downward trends; that is not their remit. It must be left to other sources to initiate research into *how* and *why* certain trends are apparent – or, indeed, why the statistics show a plateau rather than a discernible trend. The following pertinent statements and questions should be the starting point for further examination.

- Not all the health surveys gather the same data. Therefore, it is difficult to make comparisons across all four nations in terms of overall health conditions.
- In Scotland, a percentage of boys and girls were deemed 'at risk of obesity'. It is not clear what this means. Perhaps it can be construed to mean that if there is no change in their eating or physical activity habits, their weight will continue to increase at the current rate. The same report drew attention to the need to change the infrastructure, environment, culture

and social norms – but no examples were given of *how* to change them, or what is meant by some of these targets.

* It would possibly be 'nit-picking' to ask whether 'smoking' referred only to cigarettes or also to other forms of tobacco, such as cigars and pipes.
* In England, physical activity levels refer only to out of school activities. In Wales and Scotland, this exception is not stated, and in the Northern Ireland report there are no statistics under the heading 'physical activity'.
* In Wales, the survey distinguished between 'moderate' and 'vigorous' physical activity, but these categories are not defined.
* Only the English survey produced data on children's smoking habits, and not all the surveys gathered data on the use of e-cigarettes.
* Surveys, especially in London, would benefit from reporting numbers and percentages of health behaviours categorised according to ethnic groups.
* In the Welsh survey, respondents were asked whether they had eaten five fruits or vegetables on the previous day. What evidence can this provide about general eating habits?
* Only the Northern Ireland Health Survey inquired into the reasons why certain individuals gave the responses they did.

We are left with questions that need to be answered in further research, such as: Why do drinking alcohol levels in Wales increase among the higher income groups and decrease further down the income scale? Why have obesity levels in Scotland not risen over the past decade? On this last point, a recent research report from King's College, London stated that the obese in Britain represent 25% of the total population, but the numbers of those who are extremely obese continue to rise, and now stand at 500,000 men and 1.2 million women (Gimpel, 2015).

Health promotion strategies

Are health promotion strategies in the UK having any effect on combating unhealthy lifestyles, and – even more pressingly – should they bother? Contributors to Haslam and Sharma's (2014) book regret the lack of evidence that public health professionals' and politicians' efforts are positively affecting the unhealthy lifestyles of sections of the population. In this volume, Hamilton-Shield (2014, p 214) writes: 'despite numerous ... government initiatives there is still a significant section of society that seems inured and unwilling to accept the basic health message that obesity, including that in childhood, is bad for health'. In the year the book was published, there was wide press coverage of children being taken into care because their parents were considered to have allowed – or even encouraged – them to become seriously obese (Johnston, 2014).

Tackling obesity, increasing physical activity and improving diet

England

In 2001, the National Audit Office (NAO) published *Tackling obesity in England*. The statistics it presented were dramatic. In 1980, 8% of women and 6% of men were classified as obese. By 1998, these figures had nearly trebled to 21% of women and 17% of men. By 2001, 50% of women and two thirds of men were either overweight or obese, and one in five adults were obese – a number that had trebled over the last 20 years. These increases were attributed to a combination of less active lifestyles and changes in eating patterns. The four most common health problems associated with obesity were (and still are) heart disease, type 2 diabetes, high blood pressure and osteoarthritis, leading to a shortening of life by an average of nine years.

The report noted: 'halting the upward trend presents a major challenge. As a lifestyle issue, the scope for policy to effect such changes in a direct way is very limited. The Department of Health by itself cannot be expected to "cure" the problem' (NAO, 2001, p 6). Although the report called on a combination of agencies (such as the NHS, health authorities and the Health Development Agency) to address the problem of obesity, it mainly focused on GP practices. However, many GPs expressed frustration at not knowing which (if any) treatments, advice or interventions were successful in preventing or reducing obesity.

Some surgeries operated an exercise referral system – exercise on prescription – but in the majority of cases, only advice about diet and lifestyle was being offered. This advice, it would appear, is being largely ignored. According to a report in *The Times* (Barrow, 2012), campaigns to persuade the nation to embrace a healthier diet are failing. The report in *The Times* noted that a study of 3,000 adults and children suggests that there has been little change over the past 25 years. Less than one third of adults and only one in ten children eat their 'five a day' of fruit and vegetables, according to the National Diet and Nutrition Survey (2016). The same report in *The Times* noted that the Department of Health claimed there was evidence that people were heeding warnings about diet, but it would take time to have an impact on their health.

One factor influencing the increase in overweight and obesity in England was the greater availability of 'highly palatable, energy-dense foods' – presumably a reference to takeaway meals and drive-through outlets. According to the NAO report, the decline in levels of physical activity could be linked to the increasing amount of time spent watching TV and playing computer games. In addition, lack of physical activity could result from the stark difference between the amount of energy needed to carry out many occupational tasks 50 years ago and that needed to do a day's work in 21st-century Britain. Other likely causes of rising obesity levels were listed as:

- a reduction in exercise due to greater use of the car and wider car ownership;
- the decline of walking as a mode of transport because of heightened fears about personal safety, particularly in the case of children, women and older persons, and especially those living in inner cities;
- an increase in energy-saving devices, such as escalators, lifts and automatic doors.

Two other sets of vulnerable adults were people who had stopped smoking (and consequently had an increased appetite) and disabled persons.

A substantial part of the NAO report, however, stressed the importance of preventing children from becoming overweight or obese. This might be achieved through ensuring that pupils took part in at least two hours of physical activity each week and that they ate nutritional meals. Apart from health promotional measures such as these, about two hundred operations had been performed on seriously obese patients (many of which were done privately), and the government was in talks with industry to reduce the percentage of salt, fat and sugar in food and drink.

Since the 2001 NAO report, little has changed – as the most recent health survey research, summarised earlier, has shown. As in 2001, a course of drug therapy has supplemented any advice given to patients presenting as seriously overweight. A report in 2017 from the Office of National Statistics stated that pharmacies in England dispensed just under half a million weight-loss items – mainly the drug Orlistat, which prevents the body from absorbing fat from food. Two other drugs were withdrawn because they were found to increase the risk of heart attacks and strokes. Bariatric surgery was carried out in both in-patient and out-patient settings. These included gastric bypasses, stomach stapling and gastric band maintenance. In England, the number of these operations has fallen since 2011/12. A surgeon criticised this trend on a BBC programme in 2017 on two grounds: this type of surgery proved to have an immediate and lasting positive outcome, and it was effective in reducing the costs of obesity to the NHS (*How prejudiced is the NHS?* 2017). The cost-effectiveness of health promotion interventions will be addressed in Chapter Five.

Scotland

In 2010, the Scottish Government identified four key areas in which action was likely to have the greatest effect:

• reducing demand for and consumption of excessive amounts of high-calorie foods and drinks;
• increasing opportunities for uptake of walking, cycling and other activity;

- establishing lifelong healthy habits in children;
- increasing the responsibility of organisations for the health and wellbeing of their employees. (Scottish Public Health Observatory, 2010)

A follow-up report acknowledged that Scotland was experiencing an obesity epidemic, along with most of the developed world. Worryingly, Scotland had the third-worst obesity percentage of the population, behind only the US and Mexico (Scottish Government, 2016a). This report affirmed that obesity should not be viewed simply as a health issue and would not be resolved by reliance on individual behaviour change. A successful approach would require cross-sector collaboration to make changes in the living environment – from one that promotes weight gain to one that supports healthy choices: 'This is a long-term aim and will take many years to achieve. It will require systemic and far-reaching change in infra-structure, environments, culture and social norms' (p 2). The proposed 'route map' laid down the same four categories for preventative action as the aforementioned 2010 report. The success of these actions will be monitored annually.

Wales

Apart from the serious and life-threatening health risks to which obese people are prone, the Public Health Wales (2017) report adds breathlessness, difficulty sleeping, feeling tired and back and joint pain. Some people, it claims, may also experience psychological problems such as low self-esteem, poor self-image and low confidence levels, which may lead to depression. As a result, obesity can impair a person's wellbeing and quality of life. As in the reports from England and Scotland, the Wales document points to diet and sedentary lifestyle as the main causes of overweight and obesity. As in the England report, this policy document details some reasons why many people seem to make poor food choices and show a low uptake of physical activities. These include biological disposition, the supply and availability of food, advertising, changing work and living conditions (including increased use of machinery) and government policies.

All of the reports call for a collaborative approach to tackling obesity. In Wales, the policy is for the Welsh Government, health boards and local authorities to work together on an agreed agenda for change. This involves four tiers.

- *Level 1: Community-based prevention and early intervention (self-care)*
  - *Change4Life*: the social marketing programme designed to help families make changes to their lifestyles so they can eat well, move more and live longer;
  - planning policy to support physical activity and healthy eating, including active travel planning, land for growing food and location of fast food outlets;
  - community-based cookery clubs in disadvantaged communities;
  - schools adopting *Appetite for life* recommendations and developing and implementing a food and fitness policy;
  - school nurses measuring and monitoring the weight and height of schoolchildren.

- *Level 2: Community and primary care weight management services*
  - a weight management programme for children aged 7–13 and their families, which is available in all local authority areas in Wales;
  - the National Exercise Referral Scheme: a 16-week programme that enables sedentary people with a medical condition to engage in structured physical activity opportunities supervised by a qualified exercise professional;
  - identification of overweight and obesity as part of health checks in primary care.

- *Level 3: Specialist multidisciplinary team weight management services*
  - interventions such as dietary, physical activity and behavioural components delivered through primary and secondary care, which can be combined with drug therapy.

- *Level 4: Specialist medical and surgical services*
  - includes access to bariatric surgery for people who have failed to lose weight.

Northern Ireland

The Department of Health Northern Ireland (2016) report, *A fitter future for all*, was subtitled *Framework for preventing and addressing overweight and obesity in Northern Ireland: 2012–2022*. Unlike the three aforementioned documents, the Northern Ireland report set a target; namely, reducing the levels of adult obesity (including 'overweight' adults) by 4% by 2022, and reducing the levels of child obesity by 3%. Like the official statements in England, Scotland and Wales, it also recognised the types of illnesses and disabilities associated with and caused by obesity –13 in all, including mental ill health.

All four governments referred to fast food outlets and marketing of products high in salt and sugar as having a detrimental effect on health. The Northern Ireland strategies to tackle obesity and lack of physical activity are presented as three distinct tiers:

1 *universal/public health interventions*, directed at everyone in the community;
2 *selective prevention*, aimed at high-risk individuals and groups;
3 *targeted prevention*, directed at those with existing weight problems and those at high risk of diseases associated with being overweight.

A fitter future for all calls for joint action across agencies, including charities, and emphasises the need to address and tackle health issues at three life stages:

1 preconception, antenatal, maternal and early years;
2 children and young people;
3 adults and the general population.

It is the one report that highlights the importance of home economics as a school subject. It also calls on policy makers to complete health impact assessments on any relevant areas of policy making. The ministerial foreword sums up the necessary but difficult course of action faced by health promotion practitioners:

The biggest challenge we face, concerning obesity, is to change attitudes and behaviours. We must encourage people to choose to eat healthier food and to participate more in physical activity, but we must also be mindful that it should be an individual's choice to do so. People must retain responsibility for maintaining their own health and wellbeing. (Department of Health Northern Ireland, 2016, p 4)

Summary

Overweight and obesity levels have been monitored in the UK for over 30 years. During that time, much has been written in official documents about the need to stem the ever-increasing tide of an overweight population. Yet, whatever efforts have been made through 'health promotion' interventions to achieve at least a minimal reduction, they have signally failed. Interestingly, none of the four strategy documents has focused on the health perils of smoking and alcohol abuse. There has been a clear reduction in smoking habits, but hardly any progress in persuading people to drink alcohol in moderation. No evidence has been presented as to why the percentage of regular smokers in the UK has fallen over the past few decades. Smokers are still buying packets of cigarettes bearing the warning 'smoking kills' – although it could be surmised that the rising price of cigarettes, rather than any health warnings, has been the chief lever for change.

As noted in all the policy statements on health promotion, a healthier Britain cannot be achieved by enhancing 'health literacy' or disseminating advice. Many people hear, but choose not to listen. So, if tried and tested strategies to change attitudes and behaviour have proved unsuccessful, with what should they be replaced? This question will be the main focus of the book's concluding chapter. For now, it is sufficient to raise a number of lines of enquiry:

• Could potentially punitive legislation *make* people adopt healthier lifestyles? The wearing of seat belts is now mandatory. Is there hard statistical evidence that this has significantly reduced the number of traffic accidents since the legislation was introduced? Smoking in many public places and some public spaces has been banned for some years. What effect has this had on comparable rates of smokers pre- and post-legislation?

- If there is a general consensus among policy makers that people cannot and should not be influenced through health promotion projects and programmes to change their ways, should warnings be given to parents that allowing their offspring to become seriously overweight amounts to neglect, with a possible consequence of having their child(ren) taken into care?
- What action can governments take to alleviate the poor living conditions that can have a damaging effect on people's health?

On this last point, it is surely not enough to refer to changing infrastructure, the environment, culture and social norms – worthy and relevant as these aims might be. This is not to single out one passage as insufficiently precise. Too often in official policy documents, impressive language is used without defining what it actually means in practice. To have any impact on individuals and organisations with the power to bring about fundamental changes in improving health levels, politicians and health professionals need to give tangible and specific examples of how they intend to implement, monitor and evaluate innovative strategies.

For example, Andermann (2013) notes that the Ottawa Charter recognised that people's behaviours are largely influenced by their physical and social environments, and that these therefore need to be restructured, rather than telling people what they should and should not do. People do have some responsibility for their actions – but according to the Charter, health is also determined by the health of their family, their community and by broader society. To what end, and in what way, these environments are to be restructured remains unanswered.

A report by Boyce et al. (2008) set out the results of three seminars on the effects of several health promotion initiatives. A number of case studies in various parts of England, and one in Wales, demonstrated a wide range of projects aiming to change people's health-related behaviours. These included attempts to reduce smoking and alcohol misuse and to persuade people to eat a healthier diet. One recommendation was to encourage GPs to take a more active role in promoting healthy lifestyles. Another recognised the role that pharmacists could play in giving customers information and advice. After examining the results of a range of health promotion programmes and projects, the authors concluded:

> There, however, is little systematic evidence to help determine which interventions or combination of interventions are most effective in changing which behaviours and with which population group. This scarcity of evaluation data makes it difficult for commissioners to use evidence-based approaches to health improvement. (Boyce et al., 2008, p 33)

They add that many evaluations only measure the short-term effects of interventions, as noted in Chapter Three.

Smith and Foster (2014) note an apparent paradox regarding the impact of alcohol on health, posing the question: Why should some groups experience alcohol-related harms despite consuming less alcohol? The question arises because statistics indicate that even though people in the lower socioeconomic bracket consume less alcohol than those in the higher bracket, they are more likely to fall victim to alcohol-related diseases. For example, the figures quoted in the Marmot Review of Health Inequalities (Marmot, 2010) show that alcohol-related hospital admissions were 2.6 times higher among men and 2.4 times higher among women in the 20% most deprived areas compared to the 20% least deprived areas. However, as far as public health interventions are concerned, Smith and Foster (2014) reported: 'Public health interventions which rely on individuals to change, such as public education campaigns, are likely to increase health inequalities while more "upstream" public health interventions, such as price increases and restrictions on the availability of health-damaging products are most likely to help reduce inequalities' (p 7). In addition, several studies have shown that a rise in social welfare spending is associated with a decrease in alcohol-attributable mortality, whereas rising health care expenditure is not (for example, Probst et al., 2014).

Concluding thoughts

The health surveys and government policy statements summarised in this chapter demonstrate the clear commitment of all four constituent parts of the UK to improve the nation's health. The motivations for them to take on this responsibility will be discussed in Chapter Five. If there is compelling evidence that the 'social determinants of health' perform a crucial role in creating health inequalities, then it is probably beyond the capability of most health promotion projects to contribute to minimising, reducing or eliminating those inequalities. It then falls on those in power to take the appropriate action.

Cragg et al. (2013) detail a wide range of options open to a government to address the 'social determinants'. These are:

- *Material measures*: Material deprivation could be challenged through social policies, such as redistributive cash transfers to those living in relative poverty and the provision of high-quality social housing for those who cannot afford it through the private market.
- *Health impact assessments*: to assess the impact of public policies on health.
- *Social support*: interventions aiming to empower people and reduce stress in the workplace.
- *Radical politics*: In the extreme, this could involve the overthrow of capitalism, but more feasibly it might involve reforms to voting systems and more direct democracy.
- *Antidiscrimination policies*: to ensure that people with chronic health conditions and disabilities can find employment and be supported in work and the community.

Dixey et al. (2013) offer another formula for constructing government options, some of which have already been introduced in the UK:

1 *Do nothing*, or simply monitor the situation.
2 *Provide information*: Inform and educate the public; for example, as part of campaigns to encourage people to walk more or eat five portions of fruit and vegetables per day.
3 *Enable choice*: Enable individuals to change their behaviours; for example, by offering participation in an NHS 'stop smoking' programme, building cycle lanes or providing free fruit in schools.
4 *Guide choice through changing the default policy*: For example, in a restaurant, instead of providing chips as a standard side dish (with healthier options available), menus could be changed to provide a healthier option as standard (with chips as an available option).
5 *Guide choice through incentives*: Regulations can be offered that guide choices by fiscal and other incentives; for example, offering tax breaks for the purchase of bicycles to travel to work.
6 *Guide choice through disincentives*: Fiscal and other disincentives can be put in place to influence people not to pursue certain activities; for example, through taxes on cigarettes or discouraging the use of cars in inner cities via charging schemes or limitations of parking spaces.
7 *Restrict choice*: Regulate in such a way as to restrict the options available to people with the aim of protecting them; for example, removing unhealthy ingredients from foods or removing unhealthy foods from shops or restaurants.

Items 2, 3 and 6 are part of schemes in England, Scotland, Wales and Northern Ireland, and number 7 has been imposed in many schools with vending machines. Dixey et al. (2013) have labelled these provisions as examples of **advocacy**. In the context of public health and health promotion, they describe this strategy as 'a process of support for health programmes and healthy public policy ... Ultimately, advocacy in relation to policy is about trying to influence the policy-making process so that healthier legislation and healthy public policies are introduced and implemented' (p 68).

It is perhaps somewhat ironic that, mainly as a result of medical research, outstanding advances have been made (and continue to be made) in healthcare towards eliminating diseases and transplanting healthy parts of the human body in human beings with life-threatening illnesses. Yet the scourges of modern and economically wealthy countries that are often brought on by unhealthy choices continue to frustrate attempts by governments and health professionals to eliminate them. Whereas drugs and surgical procedures can alleviate and cure, health promotion has yet to find an agreed strategy to build a healthier nation.

FIVE

Health economics and health promotion

Defining terms: economics and health economics

In an era in which there is huge pressure on the National Health Service (NHS) to meet increasing demand with decreasing resources, the role of economists is central. The volume of demand has been brought about mainly because of two factors: advancements in health technology and an ageing population. As noted in the previous chapter, unhealthy lifestyles are contributing to unwelcome health conditions such as coronary heart disease, certain cancers and type 2 diabetes. With pressure to increase the NHS budget to help deal with this increase in demand, there are also concerns about whether significant resources would actually provide an improvement in the quality and effectiveness of health services. One estimate, for example, claimed that up to 25% of all healthcare services may be unnecessary (Borowitz and Sheldon, 1993), while a more recent report warned that the NHS was wasting billions of pounds because of a severe lack of efficiency (ONS, 2004). These figures need to be and will be updated later in this chapter. They suggest that the prediction made soon after the inauguration of the NHS – that within a short space of time, demand on the NHS would stabilise – has proved to be wildly optimistic.

In a speech to the House of Commons, Aneurin Bevan (1949) made this statement concerning initial anxieties about the ability of the NHS to respond to an unexpected demand for dental services and free spectacles: 'When the first rush was over the demand would even out. And so it proved. Indeed, it was proved even beyond the expectations of those of us who had most faith in the Service'. However, in a speech to the House of Commons six years earlier, Bevan had to convince opposition members of parliament to agree a supplementary estimate to the budget to increase the remuneration of student nurses.

This demand, he asserted, had nothing to do with the result of any maladministration or excessive bureaucracy. Then, as now, politicians and health professionals 'have a duty to establish not only that they are doing good, but that they are doing *more* good than anything else that could be done with the same resources' (Williams, 1993).

The discipline of economics is therefore of consummate relevance to the study of health policy and NHS funding. Economics has been defined as being founded on the premise that there will never be enough resources to completely satisfy human desires (Phillips, 2005). Consequently, government spending in one area inevitably means that resources are not available in another area. This raises a question about **efficiency** – a concept in economics that will be discussed later.

Health economics applies the principles of economics to assist in, but not wholly solve, decision-making about where and where not to allocate limited funds. Many of these decisions have to be based on consideration of other key concepts, such as **cost–benefit**, **cost-effectiveness** and **cost–utility**. Deciding where to allocate funds clearly involves not only financial considerations but also ethical questions. One of the most difficult examples is whether to spend money on maintaining a very limited life by means of a life-support machine. Another is whether to offer effective but expensive surgical procedures to prospective patients whose health problem has largely been caused through their lifestyle choices, such as heavy smoking and overeating.

Harvey (1996) revealed an interesting – and today, wholly unacceptable – view of where finite resources should be spent in the NHS. He reported that some health professionals and laypeople do not accept that resources are limited. According to this perception, the only treatments that should be avoided are those that would do harm (Kilner, 1990). A rather more justifiable position is the call for a greater proportion of the UK government's budget to be allocated to health services (Appleby, 2016). Another is the calculation that money could be saved by making sure ineffective or even harmful medical interventions are not repeated. This phenomenon, known as **iatrogenesis** ('brought on by a healer'), relates to such events as medical negligence, misdiagnosis and unfortunate but unavoidable side effects such as those resulting from chemotherapy. Illich (1974) forcefully brought the term into the health forum, but Florence Nightingale's axiom predated its essence: 'To do the sick no harm'.

Key concepts

Efficiency

Whereas economy is concerned with the costs involved in providing services, **efficiency** deals with the relationship between the inputs (costs) on the one hand and the outputs and outcomes of services on the other. In short, efficiency seeks to assess what resources are used in providing services and what the services actually produce – the ratio of total benefits to total costs. What appears to be the most economical treatment, for example, is not necessarily the most efficient. For this reason, any effort made by sections of the NHS – notably hospitals and the ambulance service – to save money might lead to inefficiency, by reducing the total benefit compared with the actual cost saved. For instance, a decision to withdraw the offer of an operation to reduce someone's level of obesity could save hundreds of pounds, but may result in an amount greater than the money saved because of continuing health promotion interventions over several years. Here is a summary of the techniques available for evaluating efficiency (Palfrey et al, 1992; Drummond et al, 2005):

- **Cost-minimisation**: Where the outcomes of two policies are identical, and there is no significant difference in the effectiveness, then the choice between policies in terms of efficiency would be made on the basis of costs, with the less costly alternative being the preferred choice.
- **Cost-effectiveness**: In many cases there will probably be differing degrees of success in achieving outcomes as well as differences in costs. The choice is then made on the basis of **cost per unit of effect** or **effects per unit of cost**. The intervention with the least cost per unit (or greatest effects per unit of costs) will be regarded as the most efficient.

- **Cost–benefit**: In most cases, it is unlikely that the outcomes of an intervention will be identical. To assess the relative efficiency, the outcomes would have to be translated, more often than not, into a monetary measure in which the ratio of costs to benefit would be compared.
- **Cost–utility**: This sort of analysis considers the impact of an intervention on an individual's and society's welfare and expresses the result in some quantitative measure. The measure is expressed in quality-adjusted life years (QALYs).

To evaluate the outputs, outcomes and impact of health promotion policies, these four criteria will need to be applied – along with more qualitative yardsticks, such as **equality**, **equity** and **accessibility**. These, as well as concepts such as 'empowerment', may be as relevant in assessing the worth of health promotion initiatives as the more quantitative aforementioned criteria listed. A potential problem in assessing health promotion programmes and projects against these qualitative criteria is finding some agreement on how these terms should be defined. For example, should 'equality' refer to equality of access to services, equality of outcome or both? To what extent can individuals with similar health needs be treated equally if, as noted in Chapter Three, they are in an experimental or control group in a randomised controlled trial (RCT)? These constitute a problem of equity.

Rationing strategies

Maybin and Klein (2012) have described ways in which the NHS can try to reduce expenditure. These are:

- **Rationing by denial:** Specific forms of intervention are excluded from the NHS on the grounds of lack of evidence about their effectiveness, high cost or a combination of both.
- **Rationing by selection**: Service providers select those patients who are most likely to benefit from interventions.
- **Rationing by delay**: The traditional form of rationing in the NHS, designed to control access to the system and try to match demand to supply by making patients wait.

- **Rationing by deterrence**: If patients are not put off by queues, there are other ways of raising barriers to entry into the healthcare system. For example, information leaflets may be unavailable regarding certain treatments.
- **Rationing by deflection**: Patients are referred to another agency, or 'difficult cases' may be transferred to another hospital or specialist.
- **Rationing by dilution**: Services or programmes continue to be offered but there are fewer nurses on the ward, doctors order fewer tests, the palatability of hospital food plunges and the quality of care and treatment declines.

The authors add that **rationing by dilution** is the least visible option, but arguably the most pervasive – and likely to become more so in hard times. On the one hand, those who defend or recommend rationing could do so according to a number of principles, such as the argument that the primary consideration should be the utilitarian ethic of maximising the health of the population. On the other hand is the argument that there is a moral obligation to cater for the health needs of individuals.

Rationing by selection has a long history. As Harvey (1996) has noted, doctors have often made a choice between patients according to criteria relating to cost-effectiveness. The simplest example involves the actions of clinicians in wartime, where the practice of triage selects those patients for whom immediate intervention can produce the most benefit. Other potential patients are left, either because they will not suffer from delay or because there is little hope of a cure. The same practice of triage obtains today in accident and emergency hospital departments; some cases categorised as nonurgent might spend prolonged periods waiting for treatment.

The population-health-maximising principle of resource allocation focuses on comparing the benefits yielded by different interventions. To this end, the techniques of cost–utility or cost-effectiveness analysis will be applied. Here, the crucial question is not whether the resources allocated to a particular individual would or would not improve the health condition, but whether the same resources would produce an even bigger improvement in, for example, a health promotion programme.

In the words of Maybin and Klein (2012, p 6), 'Population gains trump individual gains'. This principle of following the cost-effectiveness route is, according to Williams (1992), a moral imperative. The challenge of any exercise to reduce the costs of healthcare provision is to find the most ethically acceptable way to compare the benefits of different interventions. To date, the standard measure is the QALY.

QALYs

A QALY is the unit of measurement used to compare the cost-effectiveness of different treatments for the same condition. There are two components:

- the length of life in months or years that the patient can expect following treatment;
- the quality of life, measured on a scale of 0 (death) to 1 (perfect health).

The scale takes into account mobility, pain or discomfort, anxiety or depression and the ability to pursue the usual activities of daily living. This is the measure the National Institute for Health and Care Excellence (NICE) uses to make recommendations for different drugs and other treatments. An example of how the benefit would be calculated can be seen from this notional case:

> An individual with a life-threatening condition may have a life expectancy of one year with a quality of life score of 0.4 if continuing with existing care or treatment. If, however, a new drug is introduced the life expectancy is predicted to rise to 15 months with a quality score of 0.6. The old score is $1 \times 0.4 = 0.4$ but the new score is 1.25×0.6 which is 0.75 - a gain of 0.35 additional QALYs. The cost of the new drug is then fed into the calculation and the difference between this and the cost of the current treatment is divided by the QALYs gained. (Maybin and Klein, 2012, p 21)

While this quantifiable measure of comparable interventions might appear highly rational, NICE's final decision as to whether any particular drug should be introduced rests not on any strict yardstick but on an assessment of whether the cost per QALY is acceptable. In short, the limits on the threshold of acceptability are essentially 'arbitrary, based on neither theory nor practice' (Maybin and Klein, 2012, p 11). In addition, use of the QALY as the gold standard for deciding on healthcare spending priorities has been criticised for a number of reasons:

• It takes no account of the benefit that an intervention could bring to a patient's family, or even employer.
• It is not able to compute the benefit, in terms of the mental and emotional outcome, of a particular treatment or programme.
• It could discriminate against disabled people when assessing the quality of life following a treatment or nonmedical intervention.
• Some individuals rate some health states as worse than zero (death). (Coast et al., 1996; Phillips, 2005)

The notion of efficiency – which relies on calculating the cost-effectiveness of various treatments – also has its opponents, who would argue that a more important criterion affecting a judgement on where to allocate finite resources is **equity**. Should, for example, funding decisions be made that favour disadvantaged individuals and sections of the population? This would help to combat a key problem that many health promotion programmes are striving to address; that is, the problem of health inequalities. In the same vein, should resources be channelled more effectively by concentrating on the health of younger people rather than the elderly? Could NICE calculations be appropriate in comparing investment in less costly prevention policies, rather than on treatments? Considering the relatively minuscule proportion of NHS expenditure assigned to public health (which will feature later in this chapter), can a case be made for redirecting a percentage of funding from primary and secondary care into health promotion projects?

Le Fanu (1994), a general practitioner (GP), dismisses health education and health promotion as worthless activities. In his opinion, the resources put into funding these sorts of programmes and projects should be reallocated to primary and secondary health care. The title of one of his edited works is telling: *Preventionitis: Exaggerated claims of health promotion* (LeFanu, 1994). Cohen and Hale (2003) also dispute the need for the possible advocacy of health promotion as a means of providing more cost-effective programmes:

> A belief that health promotion will reduce health care costs has led many to see health promotion as a way of saving money, and economics as the discipline to highlight where these savings can be made. This shows a lack of understanding both of the objectives of health promotion and of the role that economics can play in the pursuit of these objectives. (Cohen and Hale, 2003, p 112)

Hale would agree that the objective of health promotion is to reduce morbidity and mortality, not to save money (Hale, 2000). Indeed, as Wonderling and Karnon (2010) have asserted, 'If a health promotion programme results in people living healthy lives then, in the medium term, health service costs are reduced because fewer people will be contracting diseases. But in the long term there may be no cost savings because people are living longer and consuming additional health services' (p 77). To weigh the comparative advantages of a treatment or therapeutic process against a health promotion programme could prove extremely difficult, if not impossible. As Berridge pointed out: 'Historical evaluation of health promotion cannot tell us what works best, what is cost-effective ... or advise us on the best technique for assessment' (Berridge, 2010, p 22).

Hale, however, argued that for economic appraisal to be used more widely in health promotion, the language barrier created by jargon must be eliminated. She takes as an example the economic notion of **cost**. Since resources are scarce, a cost is incurred whenever a resource is devoted to any particular use, in the form of a benefit forgone by not having used it in an alternative way.

The term **opportunity cost** is used to emphasise this notion of an opportunity forgone. For this reason, any input into a programme involves a cost, even though the staff involved are just 'doing their job'. Hale advises that this type of misunderstanding needs to be overcome, as it makes it difficult to compare the cost-effectiveness of health promotion with other health care programmes. Another salient point Hale makes is that many economic evaluations are carried out in a very specific context; therefore, care must be taken before generalising the results to other contexts or situations. The success of any programme is likely to be determined by local factors and situations, which are difficult to model and replicate.

One particular instrument used by health economists is **conjoint analysis** (another example of jargon, but its meaning is straightforward). This technique originated in the field of marketing, in which prospective buyers are presented with a number of characteristics of a particular product or service, including the cost. Respondents are then asked to rate each attribute according to their perception of its importance to them. For example, before a new model of a car is to be launched, market research participants might be asked to rate the car's fuel consumption; maximum speed; colour; design, seating and boot space. The composite results would provide helpful information towards the ultimate production of that model. Health professionals could use a parallel approach when designing a particular health promotion intervention. Indeed, such approaches have been used in health promotion for a number of years (Spoth, 1989; Spoth and Redmond, 1993); however, from public health surveys reports in the UK, it is not apparent that such preparatory work has gone into devising health promotion projects in recent years.

There might be an opportunity to introduce a more participatory approach to health promotion practice through this form of market research. As in other aspects of health policy, asking people which form of therapy or treatment they would prefer, and for what reasons, raises the question of whether all options would be available if there was a consensus of opinion about a particular preferred intervention. Another consideration is whether all the options have been subjected to rigorous testing to compare effectiveness and costs. There might well be a majority in favour of one form of health promotion that is extremely likely to be ruled out because of what is regarded as a prohibitive cost. To be upfront and honest about the likelihood of this is essential. The fact that relatively few health promotion programmes have produced unequivocal evidence of effectiveness, mainly because of the length of time needed to evaluate the outcomes and impact, is preventing a conjoint analysis approach. Ideally, it would be possible to consult the public as to which weight-loss health promotion project they would rate most highly. Should the sample of respondents be confined to individuals who wish to lose weight, or should the consultation be carried out on a sample of the public at large?

The public–at–large group might select the option to do nothing, if a significant percentage of those in the sample felt they had no need to lose weight. They could hold the opinion that scarce health resources should not be spent on people who, in their opinion, brought this health problem on themselves. Alternatively, many of the individuals in the overweight group might not *want* to lose weight. In this case, it would be appropriate to apply the economist's notion of **opportunity cost** to explain this reaction. In terms of costs and benefit, the 'cost' of following a dietary plan for a few months – where cost equals time spent buying the recommended food, or going without the much more palatable food – might or might not be worth the 'benefit' of the weight loss. The health practitioner would then face the challenge of whether to pay more attention to the 'do nothing' sample if they were in the majority. This ethical and practical situation results in criticisms of health promotion and health education (referred to in Chapter One) for attempting to impose more healthy lifestyles on certain sections of the population.

Costing unhealthy lifestyles

Despite the warnings of economists such as Cohen and Hale (2003) about the fallacy of viewing health promotion as a money-saving option, the only major rationale for supporting preventative initiatives has been its lower cost.

Obesity

Estimates have clearly shown that obesity imposes a significant economic burden on the NHS and (because of the aforementioned opportunity costs) other government functions. For example, in 2002, the direct plus indirect cost of obesity and overweight in England was £6.6–£7.4 billion (Webber, 2006). Ten years later, the Chief Executive of the NHS in England stated that the £16 billion per annum spent on the direct medical costs of diabetes and other conditions related to being overweight or obese was more than the amount spent on the police or fire services (Hughes, 2016).

One economist, however, has recently challenged these calculations (Tovey, 2017). He estimated the annual savings that overweight and obese people bring UK taxpayers by dying prematurely. Tovey points out that ignoring these savings leads to a substantial overestimation of the true burden of a high body mass index (BMI) to the taxpayer. His estimate of the present value of pension, healthcare and other benefit payments avoided through early BMI-caused deaths is £3.6 billion per annum. The net cost, therefore, is calculated as £2.47 billion, which is 0.3% of the UK's total budget in 2016 or 1.8% of the NHS budget in the same year. These figures are based on an estimated 7.1% of deaths attributed to elevated BMI in England and Wales in 2014. Each individual lost 12 years of life on average. One counterargument to Tovey's position is that if a health promotion or other intervention managed to improve the health of overweight or obese people, this could have the effect of enabling them to continue in or to gain employment, and thus contribute to the UK economy through taxation. Tovey (2017) concludes his economic analysis by criticising those who have consistently overestimated the financial burden to society of overweight and obese people as contributing to a stigmatising of those individuals, many of whom have taken to overeating because of childhood psychological traumas.

Smoking

Computing the net cost and net benefit of smoking in the UK is probably as complex as calculating the same statistics for obesity. According to a report by O'Brien and O'Leary (2015), the tobacco industry yields about £12 billion in direct tax revenue per annum. This does not include tax paid by employers of those working in the tobacco industry. The authors estimate that the costs to the NHS in any given year are likely to fall between £3–6 billion for treatment, including the cost of hospital treatment and GP and nurse consultations. In the longer term, as with obesity, the total cost might be lower, since some people who die prematurely due to smoking might otherwise have gone on to cost the service more money as a result of other health conditions and loss of productivity. The government also spends part of the budget putting out fires caused by cigarettes.

Alcohol

The Institute of Alcohol Studies (IAS) has stressed that calculating the cost to society of alcohol use and misuse is difficult. One problem is that there is significant debate around which types of cost to include. The lack of a definitive set of criteria means that there is no single figure representing the cost of alcohol consumption in the UK (IAS, 2016). In economists' terminology, costs and benefits can be classified as **private** or **external**. Private costs and benefits are those that accrue to drinkers themselves; for example, the pleasure the drinker gains from drinking would be termed a private benefit. This terminology could also, of course, apply to the benefits gained from smoking or from overeating. Private costs include the suffering associated with ill health or negative effects on earnings. External costs and benefits represent the effects of a person's drinking on others. External costs include concerns such as violence and crime caused by drinking, or the cost of treating health problems incurred as a result of drinking. Standard economic theory proposes that external costs should be reflected in alcohol taxes so that consumers bear the full social cost and not just the private cost. As with attempts to cost the economic effects of smoking and obesity, it is also relevant to compare alcohol tax revenue with public spending on alcohol-related problems, which impinge on the health system, the criminal justice system and the economy. On this last point, a study by the National Social Marketing Centre (2016) estimated that the total social cost of alcohol to England at 2007 figures was £55.1 billion, including £3.2 billion to public health and care services. Income was estimated at around £46 billion per annum.

Is prevention better than cure?

The apparent confusion – even among health economists – as to how to accurately calculate the respective costs and benefits relating to preventable illnesses prompts another question: Is there evidence that health promotion policy, centred on preventing poor health conditions and improving the prospects of people living a healthier lifestyle, is worth the investment by governments? If there *is* such evidence, should public health resources be enhanced by reallocating funding from primary, secondary and tertiary care to health promotion strategies?

In a paper published in 2008, Srivastava (2008) confronted the issue of whether public health policies and programmes had any track record of success. Wanless (2004) had already confronted the issue by stating that the lack of information on the cost-effectiveness of population health interventions was one reason for the modest investment in public health. Most of the data in Srivastava's (2008) policy paper came from the United States, and it could be problematic to assume that the results from one country are transferable to another. While it is relatively easy to measure and identify short-term outcomes and costs for vaccinations and screening, this is not the case for other preventative measures, such as health promotion programmes: 'The summary of evidence presented indicates that some prevention measures may be cost-effective but evidence on whether they lead to reduced total health care costs in the long run is not there' (Srivastava, 2008, p 10).

At this point it is important to explain that **prevention** can be interpreted in three ways:

- **Primary prevention** aims to prevent disease before it happens. This might be done through health education sessions or leaflets in hospitals and GP surgeries pointing out the risks of contracting certain diseases or disabilities. Advice may be given on the need for physical exercise, a healthy diet and moderate alcohol consumption. Other methods would be screening processes, regular check-ups for blood pressure and cholesterol levels and annual vaccinations against flu.
- **Secondary prevention** focuses on reducing the impact of a disease or poor health condition. The approach here is to set up processes that are able to detect and treat a health condition as soon as possible to halt or slow its progress. This would occur, for example, as a result of some of the primary prevention processes, such as screening and regular health checks.
- **Tertiary prevention** helps people to manage long-term, often complex health problems to improve as far as possible their ability to function, quality of life and life expectancy. This could include cardiac or stroke rehabilitation programmes, the management of diabetes, arthritis, depression as well as vocational rehabilitation programmes to help people retrain to return to employment. (King's Fund, 2017b)

It would seem that attempting to put an accurate figure on the longer-term effects of a health promotion project intended to prevent ill health or improve current health status is fraught with difficulty. Srivastava (2008) cites the example of someone engaging in physical activity who, for this very reason, might suffer an injury that will need some kind of clinical intervention in the future. One might ask how it would be possible to predict (a) the likelihood of this happening within a particular period of time, and (b) the resulting cost of treatment, particularly if the type and seriousness of the injury could not be known. The author advocates that researchers should focus on calculating the cost-effectiveness of preventative measures, not just cost savings, on the grounds that a health promotion project may be more costly but more effective than an existing programme or clinical intervention. In addition, more attention should be paid to influencing the food industry to produce healthier food items, and to ameliorating some of the social determinants of poor health and lifestyle. Finally, the report by Srivastava calls for improvements to the quality of evidence. This will require developing some consensus on the most effective analytical techniques, and stronger adherence to health economic guidelines.

Masters et al. (2017) carried out a systematic review of research articles on the return on investment (ROI) of public health interventions in a number of countries. Their final sample amounted to 52 articles. They also analysed the cost–benefit ratio (CBR). The reported ROI and CBR varied widely. The study revealed that health protection and legislative interventions generally yielded high ROI, such as a vaccination or a new tax. In contrast, interventions for health promotion had lower returns, being more complex, resource-intensive and sustained. Masters and colleagues acknowledged that the quality of the economic evaluations in the studies varied considerably, and that designing such studies can be challenging, as public health interventions are often complex and multifactorial. It can be difficult to isolate an effect size, even within an RCT: 'Some of the published literature may therefore systematically overestimate or underestimate the ROI of interventions, and hence the need for more research' (Masters et al., 2017, p 7). Nevertheless, the review concluded that certain public health interventions are cost-saving to both health services and the wider economy. Some – such as falls prevention – provide a rapid return, as do immunisation, smoking cessation and nutrition. Attempting to quantify returns within a short period can be problematic; larger returns on investment were seen over a 10–20-year horizon.

Writing within the context of the New Zealand healthcare system, Richardson (2009) listed a number of health promotion initiatives that had proven cost-effective in several countries:

- **tobacco control** through increasing unit costs, creating smoke-free environments, mass media campaigns and school education programmes;
- **immunisation programmes** in childhood against diphtheria and tetanus, and in adults against HIV/AIDS and hepatitis;

- **workplace health promotion programmes**, which reduce absenteeism.

Expenditure on the NHS

England

The latest figures, reported in 2017, show that the total budget stood at £120 billion. This amount was expected to rise by £5 billion by 2020, taking inflation into account. The government was asking the NHS to find £22 billion in savings by 2020 to keep up with rising demand and an ageing population. The official figures do not include spending on public health and training; public health spending is expected to fall, despite the need to continue and improve access to social care and place greater emphasis on prevention. About two thirds of NHS trusts, which provide secondary care for patients referred by their GP, are in deficit. In 2015–16, this amounted to £2.5 billion, and looked set to increase (O'Leary, 2017).

Between 2009/10 and 2020/21, the anticipated increase in the budget is expected to rise by 1.2% – far below the long-term annual increase (from 1949/50 onwards) of 3.7%. Unfortunately, Bevan's hope of a levelling off in demand is not forecast to happen. Instead, demands for services are expected to continue to increase. When the NHS was launched in 1948, its budget was £437 million, which is comparable to £15 billion in today's money. In 2014/15, the Department of Health allocated around £5.8 billion for public health spending. Just over £1.9 billion of this was given (via Public Health England) to the NHS for services such as vaccination, screening and health visiting. £2.8 billion was ring-fenced and allocated to local authorities as a grant, with more than half of this going on sexual health and drug services and the rest for other services such as tobacco control, obesity and physical activity (King's Fund, 2017b).

Scotland

In 2015/16, the total Scottish health budget was £12.2 billion – 40% of the Scottish Government's budget. Although the budget increased by 2.7% from the previous year, it is not keeping up with growing demand and the needs of an ageing population (Audit Scotland, 2016). The NHS boards found it difficult to achieve the savings required, and this will be even more so in 2016/17.

- £10.4 billion was allocated to the NHS boards that serve each area of Scotland and deliver frontline health services.
- £1.3 billion went to Healthcare Improvement Scotland, the Mental Welfare Commission and the seven special NHS boards that provide specialist and national services, such as the Scottish Ambulance Service.
- £0.5 billion went to national programmes, such as immunisations, health and social care integration, health improvement and health inequalities.

Between 2008/09 and 2015/16, the total health budget increased by 16% in cash terms. Taking into account inflation, the real-terms increase was 5%. The 2.7% increase included a 3.2% increase in the revenue budget – staff costs, medical supplies, rent and maintenance. Over the past five years, the annual increase has been less than the UK rate of inflation. Spending on drugs is expected to rise by 5–10% each year. The Scottish Government forecasts that the overall health budget for 2016/17 will increase by 5.6% to £12.9 billion (Scottish Government, 2016b).

Wales

The Welsh government statistics for 2015/16 showed a total expenditure of £5,802 million for the NHS in Wales. This was 4% higher than in the previous year. The largest spending category was mental health, which represented 11.4% of the total budget. One of the categories was 'healthy individuals', which included screening services and the costs of prevention programmes. Spending under this heading amounted to £109,168 (1.9%). Other Public Health Wales functions included health improvement at 1.3%.

Northern Ireland

The Northern Ireland Executive's (2016) spending budget for 2016/17 was £4.88 billion – an increase of 2.7% – of which public health services will have a budget of £67.4 million. This amounts to 1.4% of the total Northern Ireland budget. The Northern Ireland document is explicit in its commitment to public health:

> A key aim of the entire health and social care system in Northern Ireland for 2016–17 will be to improve the overall health and wellbeing of the population and to prevent ill health. This means supporting people to take control over their own lives, and enabling them to make health choices about how they live their lives. It also means working with other partners to tackle the root causes of ill health and reduce health inequalities. The health and social care service has an important role in addressing this, but it cannot do so in isolation. It will therefore work with partners across the government and other sectors in 2016–17 to address the social, economic and environmental factors that impact on people's health and wellbeing. (Northern Ireland Executive, 2016, p 72)

This budgetary statement marks Northern Ireland as the only UK nation to have overtly committed to emphasising preventing ill health, improving health and (with partners) attempting to tackle the social determinants of health. However, like the other nations' documents, it does not predict an increase in the public health budget to realise these aspirations.

Clearly, there are constraints on spending throughout the NHS in the UK. For this reason, a particular component of the health system's many clinical and community-based activities would require compelling evidence to make a claim for increased funding. To provide a carefully researched rationale for investing in public health generally, and health promotion activities in particular, NICE (2011) organised a number of workshops attended by key stakeholders in health and social care in different parts of England.

Results from the NICE workshops

The title of the workshops and the subsequent report spelled out their intentions: *Supporting investment in public health: Review of methods for assessing the cost-effectiveness, cost impact and return on investment* (NICE, 2011). The report provides guidance on how to decide whether to invest in public health initiatives and what criteria to use in reaching a decision. NICE uses cost–utility analysis, using QALYs, to assess whether or not public health interventions offer value for money. **Cost impact** is the assessment of the net costs (or savings) arising from implementing the guidance recommendations for the purpose of informing budget-setting. Cost impact considers the impact on healthcare budgets for both one-off and recurring costs within a defined time period and for a defined population.

The report clearly states the purpose of economic evaluation, which is to compare the costs and consequences of alternative courses of action. The cost-effectiveness of an intervention or programme is assessed to ensure maximum health gain from the available resources, which are finite.

> If resources are used for interventions that are not cost-effective, the population as a whole gains less health benefit (that is, there is a greater opportunity cost). However, a balance must be struck between efficient allocation of resources on the one hand and an equitable allocation of those resources on the other. (NICE, 2011, p 34)

Workshop participants were asked to rank 14 criteria in order of usefulness in deciding whether to invest in a particular public health programme or project:

- cost of intervention
- effectiveness
- cost-effectiveness score

- population eligible
- impact on health inequalities
- burden of disease
- cost saving in less than five years
- cost saving after five years
- acceptability
- affordability
- feasibility
- quality of evidence
- certainty
- non-health effect (benefits in health and other public sectors; for example, education, criminal justice)

Needless to say, there was no unanimous rating of each of these criteria, but it was instructive to record the differences. For example:

- Local authority (LA) participants ranked *health inequalities* more highly than health sector participants (first versus fourth).
- LA participants ranked interventions that are *cost saving in less than five years* more highly than those from the health sector (fourth versus ninth).
- Participants from both sectors ranked *cost-effectiveness* as the second most useful criterion.
- *Effectiveness* featured among the top three rankings for both health sector and LA participants.
- Those from the health sector ranked *affordability* more highly than LA representatives (third versus sixth).
- Those from the health sector ranked *burden of disease* more highly than LA representatives (fifth versus eleventh).

Although NICE (2011) uses QALYs as a major indicator of effectiveness, it became apparent that the QALY is too narrow to capture the value generated by public health interventions. This is because these interventions impact on a range of non-health outcomes, such as criminal justice, employment and family and caregiver outcomes. In addition, consideration needs to be given to the trade-off between the policy objective of maximising health and other gains, and that of reducing health inequalities.

The NICE (2011) guidance offers questions that should be asked when drawing up a public health/health promotion project:

- Whose health are you targeting? (age group, gender, ethnicity)
- What are the intended health outcomes? (smoking cessation, reduced weight)
- What kind of intervention do you want to be delivered? (information provision, advice, education)
- What interim outcomes are you hoping to achieve? (knowledge, availability of services)
- Which organisation(s) should provide the intervention? (NHS, LA)
- Where should the organisation(s) deliver the intervention? (primary care, school)
- Who should deliver the intervention? (GP, practice nurse, teacher)
- How should it be delivered? (one-to-one advice, small groups)
- How long should it take and how frequently? (15 minutes, 1 hour, once a week)
- Over what period? (4 months, a year)

All this guidance is intended for use as a template in designing health promotion programmes and projects. Yet there should also be some expert assistance offered on how outcomes are to be assessed, and who will decide what the outcome should be. There have been earlier references to 'empowering people' without much clarification as to what this would mean in practice, apart from empowering people to make healthy choices. This could, however, be interpreted as making the choices already predetermined by those who decide the nature and purpose of the intervention. The alternative would be to involve the intended targeted beneficiaries at every stage of the process ('targeted' to exclude the beneficiaries mentioned in the earlier discussion on QALYs' relative inadequacies).

The question 'Why?' could be added to the first question on the list above; that is: 'Whose health are you targeting and why?' It is not appropriate at this point to deal with the ethics of health promotion and evaluation; these considerations will form part of the final chapter.

Limitations of health economics

Drummond et al. (2007) identified four main challenges to those undertaking economic evaluations of public health interventions:

- measuring outcomes
- valuing effect
- incorporating equity considerations
- identifying intersectoral costs and consequences

As Marsh et al. (2012a) have noted, it is difficult to attribute change in health status to any one public health intervention (such as a health promotion programme or project) for several reasons. First of all, very few programmes would lend themselves to evaluation through the medium of an RCT, which – as previously noted – is still regarded as something of a 'gold standard' for carrying out research into the effectiveness and cost-effectiveness of health interventions. Second, many public health or health promotion projects depend on changes in individual behaviour, thus making outcomes difficult to attribute and generalise. Third, the time gap between the implementation of the intervention and the realisation of benefits, such as increased participation in exercise and its eventual positive health effects, is problematic.

Drummond and colleagues also highlight the difficulty of how to place a value on the outcome of an intervention. As noted earlier, the cost–utility approach that uses QALYs as the key indicator of a successful outcome has its limitations. For instance, a health promotion programme to tackle alcohol misuse could prove successful in reducing alcohol consumption in targeted individuals, but might also have an impact on rates of offending and improved employment prospects – neither of which can be captured using QALYs. Many public health schemes have reducing health inequalities as one of their aims, if not their principal aim. Decisions would therefore need to be made about who the targeted groups should be, and whether a higher score should be attached to an outcome that favours a disadvantaged group or individual than one favouring a more advantaged sample.

Regarding the final consideration of intersectoral costs and consequences – ultimately, the costs of interventions primarily fall on the respective departments of health within the UK's four NHS organisations. Costs will also be incurred by LAs as far as the public purse is concerned. This takes no account of certain health promotion programmes designed and implemented by third-sector organisations, particularly those concerned with mental health. These could well alleviate costs for not only the families of those with mental health problems but also employers' costs in relation to productivity and absenteeism.

The message conveyed by Marsh et al. (2012a) is that methods must be found to enable economic evaluations to go beyond traditional methods of economic analysis. Decisions about the values to be placed on nonquantifiable measures (such as satisfaction and wellbeing levels) need to be a collaborative effort, including involving key stakeholders in any specific health promotion endeavour.

Estimating costs of health promotion

Tolley's (1993) work includes a relatively early but comprehensive discussion of the different types of costs associated with health promotion, and argued that more than one type of cost needs to be considered in an economic evaluation of such activities. Which costs are included depends on the perspective of the programme. For example, a full evaluation of the costs of health promotion from a societal perspective would include all costs incurred by a range of agencies and by individuals receiving health promotion. **Direct costs** would cover the staff, materials, capital and other resources involved in the programme. If a programme of exercise-promotion sessions were to take place in a local community centre, costs would include the time of the staff member leading the sessions, any travel costs and any additional costs for using the community centre facilities. The costs to the individual participants would be the time and financial expenses of travelling to the community centre and attending the exercise sessions. Costs such as these would be eliminated if the sessions were to take place at a location usually visited by the individual, such as a workplace, unless time was allowed to attend the sessions instead of carrying out work.

There are also **intangible costs**, which would include the anxiety and stress experienced when undergoing a screening process or attending a GP surgery to have blood pressure checked. Indirect costs should only be included in an evaluation if the cost derives from participation in a health promotion programme, and not if the 'productivity losses' would have occurred anyway due to the individual's health condition.

Tolley (1993) agrees that few studies or programmes are likely to include all cost categories – especially intangible and indirect costs, which are difficult to measure accurately and reliably. An alternative approach would be to calculate the **net cost** of each health promotion option. This approach includes each of the aforementioned components but subtracts any resource savings to the health service, individual participants or other agencies – for example, reduced use of health services in the future – although this, too, would be difficult to monitor and to cost.

Another important part of any health promotion programme and evaluation of its success in achieving its objective is the method of data collection. Tolley (1993) discusses this, but it does not feature to any notable extent in the relevant literature on evaluating health promotion. Data collection using monitoring forms and diaries enables resource use to be identified as it is incurred. However, this could be time-consuming and open to possible lapses in recording an individual's participation in a health promotion activity. Alternatively, data could be collected retrospectively by means of distributing questionnaires to service providers on resources used, and to individual recipients to recall any expenses incurred.

Costs to the economy

Considering the amount of money spent on health services in Britain, the inevitable but perhaps naive question that has to be asked is: What is the point? A recent Health Foundation publication appears to provide the definitive answer: 'Good health is an asset. It is necessary for a prosperous and flourishing society' (Health Foundation, 2017, p 5). This policy document, which aims to produce a national strategy based on tackling the social determinants of health, stresses the negative impact of the loss of economic value of a workforce no longer able to participate in employment, and quotes Stickler's (2014) pronouncement that the ultimate source of any society's wealth is its people.

In a similar vein, the Scottish Government (2010b) stated: 'Attainment of the government's purpose of a flourishing economy requires a healthy population. Overweight and obesity pose real risks to the health of the population in Scotland and its ability to meet its overarching purpose of sustainable economic growth because of the burden of disease that accompanies overweight and obesity' (p 1). Northern Ireland's policy statement set out the economy and jobs initiative, which includes a number of measures to help support economic growth, including a commitment to establish a Task and Finish Group under the remit of the Connected Health and Prosperity Board (Department of Health Northern Ireland, 2014). In Wales, a Public Health Wales (2016a) strategy report placed preventing ill health and reducing health inequalities as its top priorities to achieve a number of objectives, a most important one being a sustainable economy.

Concluding thoughts

Health economists possess an armoury of techniques designed to evaluate the value for money of health promotion initiatives. To the four listed earlier in this chapter – cost-minimisation, cost-effectiveness, cost–benefit and cost–utility – others could be added, including cost-consequence and cost impact. Even this, however, would not constitute an exhaustive list. Yet, even with a wealth of economic evaluation methods, health economists acknowledge that they do not necessarily possess all the technical requirements to assess whether health promotion policies are delivering value for money.

Two crucial questions are:

- What is meant by 'value'?
- Value for whom?

There are diverse stakeholders – people looking to benefit in some way from the activity – within every health promotion project. What is not completely evident is exactly what benefit or value the promoters of the programme are hoping to derive from the project. The stated rationale for public health is to prevent ill health, improve existing health status and reduce health inequalities – but for what reason? If it is to limit the portion of the national budget spent on healthcare, that could be done overnight; it does not require the allocation of even a small percentage of the global NHS budget to public health initiatives that, on the evidence to date, rarely turn out to be unequivocally successful in achieving their stated objectives. Even the relatively few RCTs in the field of health promotion, such as the one completed by Murphy and colleagues on a national exercise referral scheme (Murphy et al., 2012), usually emerge with serious provisos about inferring any tangible cost benefits from the results.

Baggott (2000) has argued that it is by no means certain that prevention is less costly to the public purse than expanding treatment facilities. As Cairns (1995) asserted, there is very little evidence on the cost-effectiveness of prevention strategies, which often have longer-term costs that weigh heavily in the future. For example, if more people live longer because they give up smoking, this may have an impact on healthcare costs – not to mention the costs of pensions and long-term care. Richardson (2009) challenges this forecast and contends that extra years of life have value to which it is worth allocating resources. Healthcare interventions also have the potential to extend life; for example, every time a hip replacement or an appendectomy is performed there is potential for the patient to live longer and potentially develop other health problems, which will require the use of health resources.

Perhaps the 'value' is being seen to be doing something positive, on the understanding that helping people to become and stay healthy for as long as possible is universally supported as a national moral obligation. If this is true, then health promotion and health services do not entirely aim to maintain a healthy population to boost productivity and contribute to an economically healthy nation. The fact that exponents of health economics (as applied to health promotion evaluations) are critical of their own capacity to deliver hard and fast judgements might convey a message about where finite resources could most effectively be spent.

SIX

Health promotion and mental health

Introduction

Methods of dealing with the problems of mental ill-health have changed considerably in the UK over the past 200 years. The former asylums so prevalent in Victorian times were places not centred on treatment but on containment and even punishment (Scull, 2016). Today, although there are several psychiatric hospitals in the UK, both NHS and independent, the emphasis is on therapeutic approaches towards enabling patients with challenging mental illnesses to return to the community.

In England, there are three secure hospitals – Broadmoor, Ashworth and Rampton – which house individuals detained under the Mental Health Act 1983. Most of these will have been referred by the courts because of serious crimes while others are there because they are considered to be a danger to the public and/or themselves. However, since the vast majority of persons suffering from a form of mental illness pose no threat to anyone, there has been a clear shift in government policy away from hospitalisation towards investment in care in the community. Much of this chapter, therefore, focuses on public health initiatives, including health promotion, that are intended to cure or, at least to help sufferers, their families and work colleagues to cope with the personal and social consequences of mental ill-health.

Mental illness

In their book on mental illness, Ramsay et al. (2001) list the main disorders that professional and family carers are likely to face. These are:

- schizophrenia and related disorder
- bipolar affective disorder, or manic depression
- depression
- anxiety
- obsessive compulsive disorder (OCD)
- post-traumatic stress disorder (PTSD)
- eating disorders
- drinking problems
- drug misuse and dependence
- personality disorders
- mental illness in older people

Within these disorders there are subcategories. For example, there are nine subcategories of personality disorders, including paranoid (suspicious, sensitive, argumentative, stubborn, self-important) and schizoid (emotionally cold, detached, humourless, introspective); eating disorders include anorexia nervosa, bulimia nervosa and binge-eating disorders, while 'anxiety disorder' includes panic attacks and agoraphobia.

The policy that informs health promotion programmes and projects aiming to prevent disease and promote physical health focuses on what are considered the main causes of preventable illnesses: overweight and obesity, smoking, alcohol misuse and lack of physical activity. Supporting the selection of these particular health behaviours is the clinical evidence that ischaemic heart disease, certain cancers and type 2 diabetes are the direct result of unhealthy lifestyles.

Given the wide range of mental disorders and subcategories of mental health problems that may exist therein, how can those hoping to prevent or alleviate mental health problems tailor programmes to achieve the maximum benefit for their intended beneficiaries? On the face of it, it would seem an impossible task. First, there can be no specific and universally acknowledged cause of mental ill health in the generic sense that could form the basis of a health promotion intervention. Second, the outcome of a mental health promotion enterprise might be even more difficult to monitor and evaluate than a programme or project setting out to encourage, advise and support people to become healthier or remain in a fit and healthy physical state.

NHS policy

In England, the *Five year forward view for mental health* (Mental Health Taskforce to the NHS in England, 2016) reported that one in four adults in the UK would experience as least one diagnosable mental health problem in any given year. Mental health problems represent the largest single cause of disability; their cost to the economy is estimated at £105 billion a year – roughly the cost of the entire NHS. During the 1990s, according to the policy document, the Care Programme Approach emphasised the need to locate more services within the community and to devote more energy and resources to promoting public mental health. The review makes the unequivocal statement: 'Prevention matters – it's the only way that lasting change can be achieved' (p 6). It notes that half of all mental health problems have been established by the age of 14, rising to 75% by the age of 24. Children from low-income families are at the highest risk – three times that of those from the highest income bracket.

One positive factor that has emerged over the past few decades has been a more positive and accepting attitude among the public towards mental health. The report refers to the influence in this respect of Time to Change (www.time-to-change.org.uk) – a long-term project run jointly by two charitable organisations (Mind: www.mind.org.uk and Rethink Mental Illness: www.rethinkmentalillness.org.uk) and part-funded by the Department of Health – the primary objective of which is to reduce the stigma of mental illness. The 2016 *Review* is a policy statement on behalf of the NHS in England. However, numerous third-sector organisations in England are dedicated to helping people with mental health problems, a number of which are involved in health promotion projects. One of the most prominent mental health campaigning organisations is Mind. Although the 2016 *Review* was assertive in its intention to increase spending on mental health, it made no reference to the comparative spending by local authorities (LAs) in England. Mind, however, reported that LAs were spending less than 1% of their public health budget on mental health, with 13 spending nothing (Mind, 2016).

In Mind's report *Our communities, our mental health* (2016), its chief executive, accepting that 'prevention is better than cure', identified several groups of people most likely to become mentally unwell and who could therefore be the recipients of preventative initiatives. These are pregnant women; isolated people; people from Black, Asian and minority ethnic (BAME) groups, people living in rural communities and people with a long-term physical problem. Prevention strategies fell into the three stages referred to in Chapter Five – primary, secondary and tertiary – and are presented in Table 6.1.

Table 6.1: Primary, secondary and tertiary prevention strategies

Type of prevention	Stage	Target	Aim
Promotion and prevention **(primary)**	No mental health problems	Whole population and 'at risk' groups	Prevent mental health problems happening
Early detection **(secondary)**	Early stage of mental health problems	'At risk' groups and those displaying early signs and symptoms	Detect signs of mental health problems early and seek timely help
Recovery **(tertiary)**	Later stage of mental health problems	Those with mental health problems	Reduce complications of mental health problems and support recovery and wellbeing

Source: Mind (2016)

Mind's report included a number of projects aimed towards promotion and prevention and early detection. Evaluation of the projects' success in achieving their objectives produced some positive outcomes. However, the report stressed the need for more extensive evidence of the efficacy of prevention and mental health promotion projects. It recommended certain measures that should be taken to bolster the current weight of evidence. These were divided into two levels: the **individual** level, and the **organisation or societal** level. For example, a workplace wellbeing programme might assess levels of burnout or sickness absence at an organisational level. A longer-term programme might measure levels of wellbeing and mental health problems at a community level. Data collection methods included focus groups and in-depth interviews, as well as quantitative measures such as the Warwick–Edinburgh Mental Wellbeing Scale.

Scottish Health Survey

This survey, published in 2016, listed mental health and wellbeing as a key health issue in Scotland. The report stated that anxiety and depression levels were higher in the most deprived areas compared with the least deprived: anxiety at 15% compared with 7%; depression at 16% compared with 4%. The survey notes that mental disorders often coexist with other illnesses, such as cancer and cardiovascular diseases, and with other conditions, such as obesity, lack of physical activity and alcohol abuse. Statistics also show that those with mental disorders die on average 10 years earlier than the general population.

The survey followed on from the *Mental health strategy for Scotland 2012–2015* (2012). In this document, produced after wide consultation, the Scottish Government (2012, pp 15–18) set out its priorities and commitments to improve mental health services, promote mental wellbeing and prevent mental illness. These were:

- working more effectively with families;
- embedding more peer-to-peer work and support;
- increasing the support for self-management and self-help approaches;
- extending the anti-stigma agenda forward to include further work on discrimination;
- focusing on the rights of those with mental illness;
- developing the outcomes approach to include personal, social and clinical outcomes;
- ensuring that we use new technology effectively as a mechanism for providing information and delivering evidence-based services.

The strategy also included work to improve the mental health of offenders, with a particular focus on interventions to reduce offending.

Wales

The All Wales Mental Health Promotion Network (2010) estimated the overall cost of mental health problems in Wales to be £7.2 billion a year. This figure includes estimated cost of output losses to the Welsh economy. The report called for greater investment in mental health promotion, which would bring economic advantages – a consequence that features prominently in the report and in the work of Friedli and Parsonage (2009) on the situation and policies in Wales.

The Mental Health Foundation (2016b) published important statistics on mental health in Wales. Its report, *Mental health in Wales: Fundamental facts 2016,* focused on preventing mental health problems by applying a three-stage format:

1 preventing mental health problems from developing in the first instance;
2 preventing mental health problems from getting any worse by providing early interventions;
3 preventing mental health problems from having a long-term or lifelong impact by supporting recovery.

In Wales, £600 million is invested in mental health services per annum – more than any other health service funding. One of the main concerns is the increase in referrals to the Child and Adolescent Mental Health Services (CAMHS), which rose from 1,204 referrals in 2010 to 2,342 in 2014. Another cause for concern, particularly among young people, is the growing number of self-harm admissions to hospital – notably among those in the 15–19 age group. On the positive side, the proportion per 100,000 of the population committing suicide is currently the lowest in the UK – 9.2 compared with 10.3 in England, 14.5 in Scotland and 16.5 in Northern Ireland. However, the numbers of persons suffering from dementia is projected to increase by 31% in 2021, and by 44% in rural areas.

Northern Ireland

The Mental Health Foundation produced a report in Northern Ireland that was similar to its Wales report. It was slightly hampered by the comparative lack of data compared with the rest of the UK. However, some relevant statistics indicated an overall worse mental health scenario than England and, in some cases, worse than Scotland and Wales. For example, overall there was a 25% higher prevalence of mental health problems than in England. One key statistic was that Northern Ireland spends less than half of England's per capita spend on supporting people with mental health problems and learning disabilities. In 2011, spending on mental health amounted to 7% of the total health budget. Also, in Northern Ireland 80% of women have no access to specialist perinatal support, compared with 40% in England and Scotland and 70% in Wales.

As in the rest of the UK, the numbers of people with dementia in Northern Ireland is predicted to rise, from 17,765 in 2010 to 24,980 by 2021 – an increase of 41%. Suicide rates are 16.4 per 100,000 population, which is the highest in the UK. Males have a particularly high rate at 25.9 per 100,000 population. Cases of suicide are more prevalent in urban and deprived areas, while the self-harm rates are also the highest in the UK. The report notes that: 'Evidence has found that the traumatic experiences and exposure to violence related to the conflict in Northern Ireland leads to adverse mental health not only for the persons themselves, but also for their children and grandchildren' (Mental Health Foundation, 2016a, p 17). This is especially true in the most deprived areas, where 30% of persons have signs of mental health problems compared to only 15% in the least deprived. The report concludes that, as with other parts of the UK, there is an urgent need for research and data gathering on prevention and early interventions for mental health.

Physical and mental illness

The coexistence of physical and mental illness experienced by many people presents potential problems for those policy makers and practitioners intent on helping to prevent mental illness and promote healthier lifestyles. It is not surprising that someone consigned to a wheelchair for the rest of their days is subject to bouts or prolonged periods of depression due to social isolation. Conversely, a person suffering from depression might find it extremely difficult or impossible to summon up sufficient energy and motivation to engage in physical activity. These two examples of comorbidity could be multiplied many times over to gauge the prevalence of individuals in the UK suffering from both physical and mental health problems. This raises the concern for prevention and health promotion strategies and programmes as to which problem has caused the other, and therefore which to target. This is one of the key issues discussed by Armstrong (1993), who notes that there is much research evidence to show that:

- People with life-threatening, disabling or painful physical illness are at risk of becoming depressed.
- People who have good social and family relationships recover from depressive illnesses more quickly than others.
- People with psychiatric disorders have higher death rates from *physical illness*, like heart disease and cancers, than others.

On the same theme, Walsh (2011) claims that mental health professionals have significantly underestimated the importance of lifestyle factors in fostering individual and social wellbeing and preserving and optimising cognitive function. The author asserts there is considerable evidence that therapeutic lifestyle changes can be as effective as psychological therapies in improving mental health. These include exercise; nutrition and diet; time in nature; relationships; recreation; relaxation and stress management, religious or spiritual involvement and service to others. The problem of comorbidity, when a person is experiencing both physical and mental health conditions, needs greater recognition. Mental health problems are more common in people with a physical illness than among the physically healthy (Hodgkiss, 2001). For example:

- One in ten of all inpatients are confused, either in the short term (when this is known as 'delirium') or in the long term (when it is known as 'dementia'). The elderly are particularly prone to both delirium and dementia.
- One in 14 of all medical outpatients suffers from depression.
- In one in ten admissions to a general hospital for a physical illness, alcohol misuse is the underlying cause.

People who have enjoyed excellent mental health all their lives can develop a mental illness alongside their physical illness for many different reasons. Sometimes, being given a diagnosis such as cancer or multiple sclerosis can provoke psychological distress sufficiently serious to call for professional help. Alternatively, the physical disease may directly cause a mental illness; for example, a confused state may develop after a stroke. Any painful, long-term medical condition increases the risk of a depressed mood. Even treatment for a physical illness can lead to a mental illness. Intensive care rooms and isolation units may provoke abnormal suspicions and paranoid misunderstandings (Hodgkiss, 2001). Clearly, the stress involved in caring for a partner or relative can be overpowering; so what help can charitable organisations offer in any of the three stages of prevention?

Mental health charities

As well as the public health arms of the NHS throughout the UK, charitable organisations offer help and support, some for a specific mental health disorder. This means that, in terms of health promotion, the charities provide services at the secondary and tertiary stages of prevention; some also aim to prevent mental illness. The following list attempts to provide an accurate summary of the organisations' missions and key services.

Anxiety UK

Anxiety UK (www.anxietyuk.org.uk) was formed in 1970 and is user-led, in that its helpers have experienced or are still experiencing an anxiety disorder. The organisation provides support and help for anyone who has been diagnosed with, or is possibly suffering from, anxiety or anxiety-based depression. Help is offered in the form of information and a range of therapies relating to specific phobias. Anxiety UK funds research and delivers training and consultancy services. One of its key aims is to reduce the stigma often attached to mental illness. The charity notes that one in five people experience anxiety on a daily basis.

Centre for Mental Health

This organisation (www.centreformentalhealth.org.uk) concentrates on conducting research to bring about better services and fairer policies. In particular, it seeks to identify gaps in support services and provide evidence for change. It works with government, policy makers, service providers and commissioners to create social change, improve people's lives and save society money. Its research has shown that 20% of children in the UK experience a mental health problem between the ages of three and 11. Its main work areas are:

- *children*: aiming to improve the life chances of children through the support they need early in life;
- *criminal justice*: identifying effective methods of supporting and diverting people with mental health problems;
- *economics*: researching and analysing the costs of providing services, and their benefits to the people they help;
- *employment*: developing and promoting new ways of helping people with mental health problems to get and keep work;
- *mental and physical health*: working on areas where mental and physical health overlap, such as liaison therapy, and campaigning for parity of esteem for mental health.

Mental Health Foundation

This charity's mission is to help people understand, protect and sustain their mental health. Its central aim is prevention, on the grounds that the best way to deal with a crisis is to prevent it from happening in the first place. One preventative measure is the Eating Well project, founded on the premise that what people eat and drink affects how they feel, think and behave. The charity asserts that just like the heart, stomach and liver, the brain is an organ that requires different amounts of complex carbohydrates; essential fatty acids; amino acids; vitamins, minerals and water to remain healthy. As part of the preventative programme, the organisation has run a Peer Education Project aiming to ensure every school identifies and implements better practices to safeguard children's mental health.

Mental Health UK

Mental Health UK works across all parts of the UK. Its four founding members are Rethink Mental Illness, Support in Mind Scotland, Hafal (in Wales) and MindWise. The charity states that a mental health condition can affect many aspects of daily life – from physical health to home, work and managing money – and that the impact of poor mental health can be reduced by early intervention and support. However, according to Mental Health UK, only one quarter of those affected by depression and anxiety are receiving support. Every year, half a million people in England receive treatment for severe mental illness such as bipolar, psychosis and schizophrenia, with 3 million more receiving treatment for depression. Many more will be coping with symptoms like these, but without a diagnosis or treatment.

Mind

Mind includes some mental disorders that do not appear on the websites of all such organisations. These include postnatal depression, seasonal affective disorder (SAD), a type of depression that is affected by seasonal patterns with symptoms more apparent and more severe during the winter) and obsessive compulsive disorder (OCD). This last affliction might manifest itself through intrusive thoughts, such as being constantly aware of being contaminated by dirt or germs, or the repetition of certain thoughts or actions to prevent the occurrence of an adverse event. The charity sets out a list of possible causes of mental health problems, although it warns that for many people there will be a combination of factors. For those hoping to prevent mental illness from occurring, the list of causes may assist in designing appropriate health promotion interventions for a particular target population. The following factors could potentially trigger the onset of poor mental health:

- childhood abuse, trauma or neglect;
- social isolation or loneliness;
- experiencing discrimination or stigma;
- the death of someone close;
- severe or long-term stress;
- unemployment or losing one's job;
- social disadvantage, poverty or debt;
- homelessness or poor housing;
- caring for a family member or friend;
- a long-term physical health condition;
- drug and alcohol misuse;
- domestic violence or other abuse as an adult;
- significant trauma as an adult, such as military combat, being involved in a serious accident or being the victim of a violent crime;
- physical causes – for example, a head injury or a condition such as epilepsy;
- genetic factors – researchers are currently investigating whether there might be a genetic cause of various mental health problems.

A number of these factors are also included in various health promotion projects that aim to prevent physical health problems or improving physical health.

Rethink Mental Illness

This charity provides advice and information on a number of topics relating to mental health problems. These include access to health records; advocacy; antidepressants; anxiety disorders; borderline personality disorder, planning for prison release and work capability assessment. As well as providing information on which services are appropriate and how to access them, the organisation has 200 mental health services and 150 support groups in England. It offers psychological therapies, crisis and recovery houses, peer support groups and housing services. In addition, the charity campaigns nationally for policy change, and is a partner in the Time to Change movement.

SANE

The three main objectives of SANE (see www.sane.org.uk/ what_we_do/about_sane) are:

1. to raise awareness and combat stigma about mental illness, educating and campaigning to improve mental health services;
2. to provide care and emotional support for people with mental health problems, their families and carers, as well as information for other organisations and the public;
3. to initiate research into the causes and treatments of serious mental illness, such as schizophrenia and depression, and the psychological and social impact of mental illness.

SANE also supports fundamental neuroscience research, alongside studies into treatments and therapies. The charity works to make sure the needs of carers, family and friends are also catered for. SANE campaigns to influence mental health policy and improve services, as well as combating the stigma and ignorance that all too often exacerbate the distress that people experience.

Time to Change

This campaign began in 2007. Its main purpose is to get people talking about mental health to engender more positive attitudes among the public towards mental illness. Over the next five years, the campaign will aim to change men's attitudes towards mental health. Towards this end, the campaign aims to engage more with male-dominated workforces and to find more male champions. There will also be a more targeted work programme supporting young people and getting them to understand that mental health problems can affect everyone. The campaign is operating in Wales through the work of Mind Cymru and two third-sector organisations based exclusively in Wales: Hafal ('equal') and Gofal ('care').

In 2017, the Duke and Duchess of Cambridge, along with Prince Harry, led a team seeking to publicise the importance of supporting people with mental health problems. Their London Marathon Charity Appeal was called Heads Together. The publicity for the event noted that mental health problems lie at the heart of some of the greatest social challenges, and that fear of prejudice and judgment stops people from getting help, which can destroy families and lives. Heads Together set out to help people feel more comfortable with their everyday wellbeing. This campaign drew on the experience and expertise of eight other charities:

- *Anna Freud Centre*: This charity has existed for 60 years. It develops and delivers mental health care while campaigning for mental health services built around the needs and experiences of children, young people and their families.
- *Best Beginnings*: This organisation works to give every child in the UK the best start in life by supporting the mental health of pregnant women.
- *CALM*: An acronym for 'Campaign Against Living Miserably'. This charity is dedicated to preventing male suicide by helping men who are down and in crisis.
- *Contact*: A collaboration of leading military charities, support organisations, the NHS, Ministry of Defence, UK Psychological Trauma Society and top academics working together to make the most effective mental health support easily available to Service Personnel, Ex-Service Personnel and their families.
- *Mind*: see above
- *Place2Be*: This charity helps children facing such challenges as bereavement, domestic violence, family breakdown or neglect. It runs a schools-based counselling service.
- *The Mix*: This charity provides support for those aged under 25. Since one in ten young people feel that they cannot cope

with day-to-day life, The Mix offers multi-issue support with a particular focus on wellbeing. The organisation is the result of a merger of YouthNet and Get Connected.

- *YoungMinds*: This organisation has a very similar mission to Place2Be, in that it champions the wellbeing and mental health of children and young people and helps them cope with a range of adversities. It also provides a parents' helpline.

To this list could be added a number operating in Scotland (Support in Mind, Penumbra and SeeMe) and Northern Ireland (Action Mental Health Northern Ireland, Aware NI and MindWise). All these organisations work towards the same objectives of the aforementioned organisations: to increase awareness of mental illness, to counter stigma and prejudice and to improve the mental health of sufferers through a range of support services, advice and information. The Samaritans and Childline could also be added, both of which provide online services for those seeking help with primarily mental health issues:

- The Samaritans (www.samaritans.org) offers a three-tiered approach to supporting wellbeing. First, *self-help*, which involves keeping a diary to log one's ongoing moods, share feelings and track one's thoughts; second, *peer support* to contact online support groups dealing with anxiety, suicidal thoughts, depression and stress management; and third, *professional support* – professional online counselling.
- Childline is there to help children with a range of problems, including anxiety; panic attacks; eating disorders; bipolar; depression, OCD and schizophrenia. The organisation will also refer children to YoungMinds.

Mental health promotion

Prevention strategies

Perhaps the most obvious target for a preventative strategy is **suicide**. While all health promotion strategies seek to prevent both physical and mental conditions from escalating into a serious threat of suicide, three third-sector organisations have suicide prevention as their main objective: CALM, The Samaritans and Papyrus.

The prevention of suicide among young people is the mission of Papyrus (www.papyrus-uk.org). The organisation provides confidential help and advice to young people and anyone worried about a young person, helps others to prevent young suicide by working with and training professionals, campaigns and influences national policy. The Samaritans publishes annual suicide rates for the UK and Republic of Ireland. In 2017:

- There were 6,188 suicides in the UK.
- The highest rates were for men aged 40–44.
- Rates increased in the UK over the past 12 months by 3.8%. The rates were significantly higher in Wales and Northern Ireland, but there were inconsistencies in the process for recording suicides in these two countries.
- Rates decreased in Scotland over the same period by 1.4%.
- In the UK, female suicide rates were at their highest in a decade.
- The rate for males was three times the rate for females.

Because most of their interactions with people seeking help are via anonymous telephone conversations or online, it is difficult for these organisations to find out whether their primary objective of preventing suicides or suicidal thoughts has been successful. As noted in earlier chapters, the problem of discovering whether a health promotion programme or project has achieved its main objective is inherent in the process of health promotion. But this is often to do with the length of time an intervention takes to be subjected to a rigorous evaluation, not to the issue of anonymity. However, a personal email from CALM stated that the organisation has extensive impact monitoring in place, specifically for the helpline and webchat service; it was therefore able to track the number of suicides prevented, which was 341 in 2016.

It is also possible to prevent, or at least delay, the onset of **dementia**. The Alzheimer's Society website (2017) states that medical conditions such as diabetes; stroke; heart problems; high blood pressure, high cholesterol level and obesity in midlife are all known to increase the risk of both Alzheimer's disease and vascular dementia. It gives the assurance that anyone can reduce the risk by keeping to a healthy lifestyle – taking regular exercise, keeping to a healthy weight, not smoking, eating a healthy diet and only drinking alcohol in moderation. Maintaining social and mental activity are also recommended preventative measures. On its website, the organisation Dementia UK (2017) makes the same observations on reducing the risk of dementia. The fact that certain forms of dementia can be prevented is possibly not widely known.

There was already sufficient evidence several years ago that physical exercise could have a positive impact on a person's mental health. Reviewing a substantial number of studies, Fox (1999) investigated the evidence for physical activity and dietary interactions affecting mental wellbeing. The results showed that aerobic exercise could serve as a therapy for anxiety and depression.

National Institute for Health and Care Excellence (NICE)

NICE (2011) has produced guidelines for dealing with mental health problems, which are intended for healthcare professionals, commissioners and providers, adults with mental health problems, their families and carers. The guidelines are organised into five sections:

1 improving access to services;
2 stepped care;
3 identification and assessment;
4 treatment and referral for treatment;
5 delivering local care pathways.

There is no advice on preventing mental health problems; the content focuses on following proper procedures, and lists the main mental health conditions and their possible clinical and pharmacological treatments.

There is more of a preventative theme in NICE's guidance on mental health and learning disabilities (NICE, 2016). Important motivations for NICE writing this online document were (a) that people with learning disabilities are at increased risk of mental health problems, and (b) that mental health problems are often overlooked in people with learning disabilities. Helping to prevent the onset of mental illness, including dementia, centres on annual health checks and reviews. An annual health check should focus on:

- any change in the person's behaviour;
- any loss of skills, including self-care;
- a need for more prompting in the past few months;
- social withdrawal;
- irritability;
- avoidance;
- agitation;
- loss of interest in activities they usually enjoy.

The report states that the emphasis in any intervention should be on outcomes. To this end, any services should be regularly audited to assess their effectiveness, accessibility and acceptability.

Mental health and learning disabilities

A report by the Joint Commissioning Panel for Mental Health (2013) concerning mental health and learning disability found that in 2012, only 52% of persons eligible for a learning disability check received one. This was deemed unacceptable, since the increased prevalence of mental health problems among people with learning disabilities was 30–50%. In particular, the report found that adults with Down's syndrome were significantly at risk of developing Alzheimer's disease. It stressed the need for improved coordination between the different agencies providing services for mental health and learning disabilities. Its guidelines applied only to adults; there was no section devoted to preventative action.

The other significant contributor to research into and support for people with mental health problems and learning disabilities is the Foundation for People with Learning Disabilities, which is part of the Mental Health Foundation. The Foundation's report (2017) catalogued some key statistics:

- Children and young people with learning disabilities are much more likely to live in poverty, have few friends and have additional long-term problems, such as epilepsy and sensory impairments. All these factors are associated with mental health problems.
- People with learning disabilities display a higher prevalence of the full spectrum of mental health problems than those without learning disabilities.
- Prevalence rates for schizophrenia are approximately three times the rate for the general population.

The Foundation does not describe any particular methods used to detect the existence of mental health problems for those who have learning disabilities, or to prevent its onset.

Faculty of Public Health (UK)

In 2010, the Faculty published a detailed account of methods and projects designed to prevent mental illness. It reported on research showing that most mental illness has its origins in childhood: 'The most important opportunities for prevention of mental illness and promotion of mental health therefore lie in childhood, many of them in the context of the family' (Faculty of Public Health, 2010, p 1). The report claimed that the most important influence on a child's mental and emotional development is parenting. The key way to reduce risk in early childhood is to promote healthy parenting, focusing on the quality of parent–child relationships and parenting styles, including behaviour management. Parental mental illness and lifestyle behaviours, such as smoking and drug and alcohol misuse, are important risk factors for childhood mental health problems. Schools also offer important opportunities for mental health promotion and prevention; for example, by dealing with bullying. Targeting parents – though an attractive method of intervention, according to the report – can be inefficient because there is no reliable way to identify high-risk groups; for example, parents with mental illness or who abuse drugs and alcohol. However, some projects are delivering targeted provision, such as focusing on teenage parents and those living in socially disadvantaged areas. The report recognises the potential difficulties of carrying out research that will clearly demonstrate the success of a project: 'Many different types of research are needed to tell whether interventions, programmes or approaches make a difference, for whom, in what circumstances. Randomised controlled trials (RCTs) are often difficult to carry out in health promoting settings and, while reducing some biases, may introduce others' (p 2).

Stewart-Brown and McMillan (2010) agree with this statement, having carried out a comprehensive review of systematic reviews from many countries that aim to improve parenting skills and behaviours to prevent an adverse impact on children. Results indicated that antipoverty strategies alone will not improve parenting, but that factors that can prevent children from the deleterious effects of suboptimal parenting include educational achievement, and – most significantly – a positive relationship with at least one parent during childhood. Another finding was that maternal depression during the perinatal period interrupts mother–infant communication and has a detrimental effect on the infant's and child's mental health. The most successful interventions to prevent perinatal and postnatal depression were shown to be a cognitive behavioural approach, psychotherapy and counselling.

Locations for mental health promotion

Prisons

Adults

A report by the Prisons and Probation Ombudsman (PPO) (2016) referred to a number of studies that compared the mental health conditions of adult prison inmates with those of the general population. The review by Singleton et al (2001) revealed that under the categories of schizophrenia, personality disorder, neurotic disorder (for example depression), drug and alcohol dependency, adult prisoners were up to sixteen times more likely to suffer from a mental disorder compared with the general population. The PPO report acknowledged that the research by Singleton and colleagues carried out in 1998 was quite old and that new research was called for – particularly given that, since 1998, the prison population had not only increased but also aged. The report also noted that the prevalence of mental health issues in the prison population is considerably higher than in the general population. Distance from family and relatives or isolation could make coping particularly difficult.

According to a report by the Social Exclusion Unit (2002), compared with the general population, prisoners are 13 times as likely to have been in care as a child; 13 times as likely to have been unemployed; ten times as likely to have been a regular truant, two and a half times as likely to have had a family member convicted of a criminal offence and 15 times as likely to be HIV positive. In addition, the report recorded that 70% of prisoners were using drugs before imprisonment; over 70% suffered from at least two mental disorders, while 20% of male and 37% of female sentenced prisoners had attempted suicide in the past.

Originally, the Home Office was responsible for healthcare provision for prisoners. From 2006, responsibility was transferred to the NHS. The government had previously laid down the principle of 'equivalence' – that prisoners should receive the same level of healthcare provision in prison as they would in the outside community (Reed, 1992). However, the Ombudsman stated that, as well as a considerably higher prevalence of mental health issues, a much higher proportion of prisoners have experienced a lifetime of social exclusion. For that reason, a model of mental healthcare applied in the community was unlikely to be suitable for use in a prison without being specifically adapted to meet prisoners' needs.

In 2001, the Department of Health introduced a strategy to modernise the mental health services delivered in prisons. The strategy outlined a range of types of care that should be available in prisons, including primary care services, mental health promotion, wing-based services and day care. In addition, mental health in-reach teams were introduced into prisons to provide similar services to community mental health teams. Within the category of health promotion interventions, talking therapies take place in prisons, including counselling, cognitive behavioural therapy and anger management courses. The PPO report concludes that, where an inmate has a dual diagnosis of a mental health problem and substance abuse, there should be much better coordination between those dealing with these issues.

Parsonage et al. (2009) recommended **diversion** as an alternative to imprisonment for a large number of offenders. They argued that many people in the criminal justice system have complex mental health and other needs, which are poorly recognised and inadequately managed. Too many end up in prison – a high-cost intervention, which is inappropriate as a setting for mental health care and ineffective in reducing subsequent offending. The evidence collected by the authors indicates that well-designed arrangements for diversion have the potential to yield benefits, including:

- cost and efficiency savings within the criminal justice system;
- reduction in reoffending;
- improvements in mental health.

> There is a particularly strong case for diverting offenders away from short sentences in prison towards effective treatment in the community. Diverting people towards effective community-based services will improve their mental health. It can also reduce the prevalence of other risk factors such as substance misuse and improve the effectiveness of interventions aimed at other influences on offending. (Parsonage et al., 2009, p 5)

This suggests that health promotion programmes to prevent offenders from reoffending could play an important part in the diversion system, and Parsonage and colleagues recommend that voluntary organisations could undertake some of these programmes.

In England and Wales, the first diversion scheme was established in 1989 with joint funding from the Department of Health and the Home Office. In the late 1990s, mental health courts were set up in the US, Canada and Australia – but not the UK. Coverage remains well short of the nationwide network of diversion schemes recommended by the Reed Report (2003).

Any recommendations relating to the possible outcomes and cost-effectiveness of diversion schemes must remain tentative, in view of the relative dearth of research studies in the UK.

Reed noted that over 200 years ago, John Howard, the first prison reformer in the UK, published a volume in which he observed the very high number of people with mental illnesses in prison and the poor care they received there (Howard, 1777). He complained that no care was taken of them, although they could probably have benefited from medicines and proper regimen, and some might have been restored to their senses and usefulness in life. In 2017, NICE called for annual mental health checks for thousands of criminals and others with suspected psychiatric problems when they come into contact with the criminal justice system. It also recommended that everyone being put in a cell should first be assessed for self-harm. A record 119 inmates killed themselves in English and Welsh jails in 2016 (*The Times*, 21 March 2017).

Young offenders

Chitsabesan et al. (2006) surveyed the mental health needs of young offenders in England and Wales. Using a sample of those in custody and offenders in the community, the researchers found that both groups showed symptoms of depression; anxiety; PTSD; psychosis, self-harm and hyperactivity. In all, 31% of the total sample showed these signs, with 20% also having a learning disability. The authors concluded that the assessment of mental health needs and the promotion of young people's wellbeing within the youth justice system were integral to the delivery of effective youth justice services.

Woodall (2007) investigated exactly who should provide mental health promotion programmes and interventions within a Young Offenders Institution (YOI). There were, however, severe limitations to this study; only 15 young offenders took part in the qualitative interviews – 12 in a focus group and three individually. The study demonstrated that the masculine culture within the YOI tended to militate against the young men opening up about their feelings. Efforts by The Samaritans were criticised as largely unhelpful, with participants suggesting that ex-prisoners might make more progress in supporting the offenders while they were inside. The message from the research was that promoting health and dealing with the health needs of offenders are complex issues, and that – understandably – a YOI is not principally in the business of mental health promotion: 'Prisons are penal institutions where the main aims of imprisonment are not primarily to do with self-esteem, autonomy and empowerment, rather control, discipline and surveillance, usually in an atmosphere which generally contradicts the democratic principles of health promotion' (Woodall, 2007, p 13).

In England, Khan and Wilson (2010) carried out interviews with professionals working in 55 youth offending teams and visited youth courts. The term 'complex' also features in their account of trying to prevent initial or further offending, particularly when a large range of workers were involved. In the case of a young person identified as having mental health problems, the criminal behaviour could be a result of underlying depression, or depression could be the result of involvement in criminal behaviour and its consequences. The authors state: 'It would be wrong, therefore, simplistically to assume that addressing mental health issues will necessarily influence offending levels' (Khan and Wilson, 2010, p 18). However, they add that health and mental health inequalities and needs should be a focus for intervention, regardless of the likelihood of changing offending behaviour. The inference they draw from their study is that early identification of mental health problems and conduct disorder in young people needs to activate liaison with parents, since family breakdown and harsh or inconsistent parenting are often the causes of children's future offending.

Schools

Over the past two decades, concerns about the mental health of schoolchildren at both primary and secondary levels have increased. A report by Meltzer et al. (2000) noted the prevalence of mental health problems among children, particularly those from a poor socioeconomic background. Years later, the UK government's mental health champion for schools, Natasha Devon, criticised the approach to tackling these problems (Weale,

2016). She warned that the mental health of children was far worse than expected, and that although certain behaviours (such as alcohol and substance misuse) were decreasing, the rates of depression and anxiety had increased by 70% in a generation. What was disturbing, according to the Minister, was that there was too much focus on symptoms rather than causes. As a result, there was a danger of 'medicalising schools' (Weale, 2016). There was a need to ask: What are the emotional and mental health needs of children, and are they being met? With children as young as four years old sitting tests, and an increase in bullying on social media, a much more radical approach was needed.

Who, then, should be instrumental in recognising and helping schoolchildren with mental health problems? Loades and Mastroyannopoulu (2010) claimed that teachers' perceptions of children's mental health problems were relatively unexplored. They asked 113 primary school teachers to complete a questionnaire, composed of vignettes describing children with symptoms of a common emotional disorder and a common behavioural disorder. Subsequently, teachers were asked a number of questions regarding problem recognition and help seeking. They found that teachers were able to recognise the existence of a problem and rate its severity. They were more concerned about a child with a behavioural than an emotional disorder. The impetus for this research was that mental health problems in children increase the likelihood of poor behaviour in school, low school achievement and potentially school exclusion. The authors concluded that teachers could benefit from further training to refine their ability to identify and act on children's mental health problems in a timely manner, thus minimising the need for future intervention.

Two charities undertake further mental health promotion in schools: Place2Be and the British Association for Counselling & Psychotherapy (BACP). The former, as noted earlier, provides individual and group counselling in schools via clinical staff and highly skilled volunteers. Support is also provided for parents, while training, individual advice and support is offered to school staff.

The BACP is involved with school-based counselling and carries out research into its effectiveness. School-based counselling is received by 70,000–80,000 young people in the UK every year. In Wales, there is now a statutory duty for authorities to provide access to a school-based counselling service (BACP, 2013). The effectiveness of counselling in schools has proved positive in reducing psychological distress in young people, who regard it as non-stigmatising, accessible and helpful (Cooper, 2013). Secondary school pupils have reported that attending counselling sessions has had a positive impact on their studying and learning (Rupani et al, 2012). School staff have also reported improvements in attainment, attendance and behaviour of young people who have accessed school-based counselling services (Pybis et al, 2012; Cooper, 2013).

Although further research is called for to assess the outcomes of school-based counselling services, the evidence so far suggests that this type of mental health promotion strategy is effective. Perhaps it proves an obvious point: that wherever possible, policies and programmes aimed at early intervention have the greatest potential for success – and probably value for money – in terms of prevention.

The workplace

The Advisory Conciliation and Arbitration Service (ACAS) is very active in pursuing the interests of employees who might be suffering from a mental health problem. They recently commissioned research into the current state of employer provision for vulnerable members of staff (Hudson, 2016). The report pointed out that mental illness is the largest single cause of disability in the UK, costing employers £30 billion a year through absence and lost production. It noted that the complexity, diversity and range of root causes of mental health conditions made managing mental health at work difficult – especially for line managers, who are often on the frontline supporting colleagues or signposting them to additional support.

Several factors within and beyond the workplace were found to contribute to mental health problems in the workplace. Outside work, these included bereavement; relationship breakdowns; family problems; addiction; finance, debt and housing issues. In the vast majority of cases, such influences were acknowledged as beyond the influence and control of employers. Organisational change, downsizing, increasing workloads and pressure at work can manifest themselves in potentially negative ways. These phenomena were likely to be aggravated in an 'anxious organisation' – one that struggles to manage change effectively, is under relentless pressure to perform better and has a management culture that mirrors anxiety rather than contains it. Interviews with a sample of employees during the research provided some important considerations for employers to bear in mind after a staff member returns to work after absence due to a mental health problem. Factors that helped employees to return to work included:

• having time to access the help of health professionals, such as their own GPs and counsellors;
• not being pressurised to return to work prematurely, but instead being given time, space and a sense of control over the pace of their return to work;
• being given time to become re-orientated to the workplace;
• reasonable adjustments – for example, changes to hours of work and avoiding sources of stress that might trigger symptoms.

Under the Equality Act 2010, employers have an obligation not to discriminate against any person who has a disability, which the Act defines as a substantial and long-term adverse effect on a person's ability to carry out normal day-to-day activities. Such conditions include depression, schizophrenia, bipolar disorder and OCD.

Ten years earlier than the work of Hudson (2016), Noblet and LaMontagne (2006) were critical of a workplace health promotion approach that concentrated solely on the individual. Furthermore, they added what would seem to be an obvious missing dimension to Hudson's analysis: the workplace factors that caused some staff to suffer mental health problems, rather than just external factors. They considered the direct impact of working conditions on health and employees' ability to adopt and sustain healthy behaviours. They defined occupational stress as occurring 'when demands and conditions do not match a person's needs, expectations or ideals or exceed their physical capacity, skills or knowledge for comfortably handling a situation' (Noblet and LaMontagne, 2006, p 2). For employees, chronic exposure to stressful situations – such as work overload, poor supervisory support, interpersonal conflict and low input into decision-making – have been linked to a range of debilitating health outcomes, such as depression, anxiety, emotional exhaustion, immune deficiency disorders and cardiovascular disease. Noblet and LaMontagne (2006) also reported that stressful working conditions can directly impact employees' wellbeing by limiting their ability to make positive lifestyle changes to behaviours such as smoking or being sedentary. They recommended that those seeking to reduce mental health problems and their detrimental effect on the organisation (such as absenteeism and impaired productivity) should adopt a more comprehensive approach to workplace health promotion, addressing both individual and organisational factors. Even earlier, Chu and colleagues (2000) had stressed the importance not of drafting in external health professionals to help individuals return or remain in work despite their mental health problems, instead urging organisations to involve workers and management collectively to endeavour to change the workplace into a health-promoting setting.

Economic evaluations of mental health promotion

Zechmeister et al. (2008) questioned whether it was worth investing in mental health promotion and mental illness prevention. In particular, their systematic review of published articles concentrated on programmes to prevent depression or suicide. As with all studies carried out in a variety of countries, the results – whether positive, negative or unsure – cannot be reliably transferred to other countries because of their different healthcare systems. In England, Petrou et al. (2006) evaluated a preventative intervention targeting women at high risk of developing postnatal depression. Based on an RCT, they found a nonsignificant increase in depression-free months. The probability that the intervention was cost-effective was reported to be 70%.

Five studies in Petrou et al's review examined the economic case for suicide prevention. One study in England made a cost-effectiveness analysis of a home-based social work intervention for children and adolescents who had deliberately poisoned themselves. The researchers found no cost benefits. The study aimed to reduce suicidal thoughts and costs from future demands on services. The research found no statistically significant differences between the intervention and nonintervention groups in terms of outcome and total costs (Byford et al, 1999). Another study analysed the net benefit of two programmes: general suicide awareness, and peer support programmes for the prevention of suicides among university students in Florida. The results showed that introducing either programme in all universities in Florida would achieve net cost benefits (Sari et al., 2008).

Overall, however, only a few of the studies reviewed by Zechmeister and colleagues (2008) provided strong evidence that preventative interventions were cost-effective. The clearest evidence, albeit in a US context, suggests that early intervention programmes for children and adolescents are worth financing. Despite the commitment of the UK and other countries to preventing suicide, few studies have calculated the cost-effectiveness of suicide prevention programmes. As with other areas of public health evaluation, the principal challenge relates to the questionable attribution of effectiveness and cost-effectiveness to complex interventions with long-term outcomes. Greater investment in long-term follow-up studies is required to overcome this problem.

Clearly, if workplace health promotion initiatives result in employees (a) successfully returning to work after an absence for mental health difficulties, and (b) being prevented from experiencing mental health problems because of a health-promoting organisation, there would be discernible economic benefits for the employer. However, as with so many health promotion programmes and projects, outcome evaluation has had difficulty providing sufficiently valid evidence about whether the intervention has achieved its objectives.

The aforementioned report by Friedli and Parsonage (2009) focused on the economic case for investment in mental health promotion and preventing mental illness in Wales. It considered the costs of output losses to the economy resulting from the adverse effects of mental health problems on people's ability to work. Although, as the authors admit, there is relatively limited research-based evidence on the cost-effectiveness of mental health promotion measures, the available evidence indicates that the most cost-effective areas of intervention are likely to be:

- *supporting parents and early years*: parenting skills training/ preschool education/home learning environment;
- *supporting lifelong learning*: health-promoting schools and continuing education;
- *improving working lives*: employment/workplace;
- *positive steps for mental health*: lifestyle (diet, exercise, alcohol use) and social support;
- *supporting communities*: environmental improvements.

As noted earlier, in this context mental health problems have an adverse effect on employment and output. Friedli and Parsonage (2009) estimate that absence through sickness due to mental illness cost the Welsh economy £1,161.5 million and worklessness £1,409.6 million. The Sainsbury Centre (2007) estimated that in the UK as a whole, the total cost of mental health problems in the workplace amounted to nearly £26 billion because of sickness absence, reduced productivity at work and replacing workers who leave their job because of mental ill health.

Concluding thoughts

In view of the long history of stigma attached to mental illness and its sufferers, it is heartening to know that projects such as Time to Change are helping to turn negative views into more positive recognition and acceptance of mental ill health. In addition, the many charities dedicated to preventing mental illness and helping those affected by mental disorders (and their families) provide evidence of society's view of mental health problems as a blight that affects one in four of the UK population. The constituent governments in the UK that control the NHS within their own borders are also making efforts to raise the profile of mental health – formerly the Cinderella of NHS services – into a condition that deserves increased funding. This, indeed, was one of the main policy statements during the UK election campaign in 2017.

Unlike health promotion campaigns and policies that focus on preventing poor physical health or improving the morbidity and mortality rates of people and communities depicted as following unhealthy lifestyles, there is little evidence that mental health promotion is likely to be regarded in some quarters as a waste of money. The criticism that any efforts to educate individuals about the need to adopt less damaging lifestyles are futile has not translated into public condemnation of sufferers from mental health conditions having brought the illness on themselves. While some will argue that persons who are obese might not want or need to change their lifestyle, it is unlikely that anyone today would assume that the same attitude might exist in people suffering from a mental illness.

As with all health promotion initiatives, mental health promotion seeks to establish evidence-based approaches that will prove the effectiveness and cost-effectiveness of a range of interventions. What evidence there is indicates that early interventions, particularly those that engage with parents and parents-to-be, are most likely to prevent the onset of mental illness in children. Schools will therefore play a pivotal role as the primary location for preventative mental health promotion. Such an approach could provide an additional dimension to the concept of 'health education'.

SEVEN

International perspectives

The global picture

Health promotion is a global enterprise. Three years after the establishment of the United Nations in 1945, the World Health Organization (WHO) was founded. Its remit is to help to promote and protect health and prevent and control disease throughout the world. It does this mainly by means of up-to-date information about the prevention and treatment of diseases and disseminating this information through its publications.

Forty years after the WHO was founded, in September 1978, the First International Conference on Primary Health Care was held in Alma Ata in the USSR. The conference called on all health and development workers and the world community 'to protect and promote the health of all the people of the world' (Declaration, p 1). The declaration stated that health is a state of complete physical, mental and social wellbeing, not merely the absence of disease or infirmity, and that it is a fundamental human right. It condemned the gross inequality in health status between people in developed and developing countries, and asserted that 'the promotion and protection of the health of the people is essential to sustained economic and social development and contributes to a better quality of life and world peace' (p 1). It also called for 'the attainment by all peoples of the world by the year 2000 of a level of health that will permit them to lead a socially and economically productive life' (p 1). This target was to be attained by redirecting resources currently being committed to armaments and weapons of war to health.

Clearly, this aspiration has not been fulfilled, and several further conferences since the Alma Ata Declaration have laid down internationally approved policies to maximise health resources and greatly improve the levels of health across the globe. One of the most influential of these was the Ottawa Charter for Health Promotion, published in 1986, which will be discussed shortly.

Thomas McKeown, a professor of social medicine at the University of Birmingham in the UK, introduced the notion of the social determinants of health (McKeown, 1972; 1976). As noted in Chapter Five, by increasing access to health services the National Health Service (NHS) actually increased demand. McKeown argued that there were several influences on health apart from traditional health and medical services, and that these influences should be considered in framing health policy and in any efforts to improve the health of the population (Glouberman and Millar, 2003). In particular, he contended that population growth was due primarily to a decline in mortality from infectious diseases. This decline was driven by economic conditions during and after the Industrial Revolution, which led to rising standards of living and better food that bolstered resistance to disease. Other influences – such as curative medical interventions and sanitary reform – played only a marginal role in population change. In short, the rise in population was due less to medical efforts than to economic forces that changed social conditions.

McKeown's thesis had a significant influence on Lalonde's (the Canadian Minister of National Health and Welfare) 1974 report, which adopted the position that the main determinants of health lay outside the healthcare system. According to Glouberman and Millar (2003), the idea of health promotion grew out of the Lalonde report. This proposed health education and social marketing as the means of persuading people to adopt healthier lifestyles. It also recommended other initiatives, though, such as appropriate legislation to improve the environment.

The Ottawa Charter for Health Promotion

Canada became something of a focal point for the development of health promotion policy. In 1986, an international conference, held as a result of growing expectations for a new public health movement around the world, published the Ottawa Charter for Health Promotion. Laverack (2014) has summarised this Charter and the pronouncements of subsequent allied conferences. The conference statement defined health promotion as the process of enabling people to increase control over and improve their health. The Charter listed five health promotion areas for achieving better health:

* building healthy public policy
* creating supportive environments
* strengthening community action
* developing personal skills
* reorienting health services

These areas are briefly discussed next.

Building healthy public policy

This means policy makers in all sectors should take into account the potential consequences of their decisions on the health of the population. In today's parlance, this would be called 'health impact assessment'. What has come to be known as the 'new public health' should address economic, political and environmental targets, not limit itself to medical inputs. Thus, public health could be regarded as having returned to its roots in the Sanitary Reform Movement (Green and Thorogood, 1998). The WHO had already advocated a broader approach to tackling health problems in its report of 1986: 'Health promotion policy requires the identification of obstacles to the adoption of healthy public policies in non-health sectors, and ways of removing them' (WHO, 1986, p 1).

Creating supportive environments

Changing patterns of life, work and leisure have a significant impact on health. Work and leisure should be a source of health for people. Health promotion policies should generate living and working conditions that are safe, stimulating, satisfying and enjoyable. The protection of the natural and built environments and the conservation of natural resources must be addressed in any health promotion strategy.

Strengthening community action

'At the heart of this process is the empowerment of communities – their ownership and control of their own endeavours and destinies' (p 2). Public participation in health matters is important. This requires continuing access to information, learning opportunities for health and funding support.

Developing personal skills

Enabling people to learn to prepare themselves for all of life's stages and to cope with chronic illness and injuries is essential. This has to be facilitated in school, home, work and community settings. Providing information and education for health increases the options available for people to exercise more control over their own health and over their environments.

Reorienting health services

Individuals, community groups, health professionals, health service institutions and governments must work together in a health promotion direction rather than relying exclusively on clinical and curative services.

The Charter added eight fundamental conditions and resources for health:

- peace
- shelter
- education
- food
- income
- a stable ecosystem
- sustainable resources
- social justice and equity

The Adelaide Conference (1988)

This conference, which 220 participants from 42 countries attended, addressed the first of the five action areas set out in the Ottawa Charter: building healthy public policy. The conference affirmed that healthy public policy will lead to long-term economic benefits. It laid down four key areas for immediate action:

* **Supporting the health of women**: including support mechanisms for caring work, particularly with children.
* **Food and nutrition**: eliminating hunger and malnutrition.
* **Tobacco and alcohol**: governments to set targets to reduce tobacco growing and alcohol production, marketing and consumption by the year 2000.
* **Creating supportive environments**: public health and ecological movements to join together to develop strategies in pursuit of socioeconomic development and the conservation of the planet's limited resources. (WHO, 2009a)

The Sunsdvall Conference (1991)

This conference in Sweden addressed the second of the five action areas from the Ottawa Charter: creating supportive environments. Participants from 81 countries attended. The conference pointed out that millions of people are living in extreme poverty and deprivation in an increasingly degraded environment that threatens their health, making the goal of 'health for all' by the year 2000 extremely hard to achieve. The way forward lay in making the physical, social, economic and the political environment conducive to health rather than damaging it. Action to achieve social justice in health was urgently needed to narrow the health gap between and within nations. In many countries the population had to endure armed conflicts and to survive without clean water, adequate food, shelter or sanitation. Many women were still oppressed, sexually exploited and suffered from discrimination in the labour market. Action would involve such sectors as education, transport, housing, urban development, industrial production and agriculture.

The Jakarta Conference (1997)

The statement from this conference endorsed health as a basic human right and affirmed the five action areas set out in the Ottawa Charter. It emphasised the need for effective partnerships for health and social development and stressed that health promotion is carried out by and with people, not on or to people. Health promotion improves both the ability of individuals to take action and the capacity of groups, organisations and communities to influence the determinants of health. Empowering individuals demands more consistent, reliable access to the decision-making process and the skills and knowledge essential to effect change. To make progress towards global health promotion, the conference called for the formation of a global health promotion alliance. Priorities for this alliance included:

- raising awareness of the changing determinants of health;
- supporting the development of collaboration;
- mobilising resources for health promotion;
- accumulating knowledge on best practice;
- enabling shared learning;
- promoting solidarity in action;
- fostering transparency and public accountability in health promotion.

The Mexico Global Conference (2000)

The declaration from this conference, signed by the representatives of 88 countries, reiterated the need for stronger collaboration among a wide variety of agencies, including the private sector, and that health promotion contributed to social and economic development and to the principles of equity. The statement at the end of the conference drew attention to the need to address the social, economic and environmental determinants of health, and that this requires strengthened mechanisms of collaboration for the promotion of health across all sectors and at all levels of society. The conference concluded (a) that health promotion must be a fundamental component of public policies and programmes in the pursuit of equity and better health for all, and (b) that there is ample evidence that good health promotion strategies are effective.

The Bangkok Charter for Health Promotion in a Globalized World (2005)

A statement from this conference drew attention to changes in the global context since the Ottawa Charter. It listed some of the critical factors that now influenced health:

- increasing inequalities within and between countries;
- new patterns of consumption and communication;
- commercialisation;
- global environmental change;
- urbanisation.

Other factors to be taken into consideration included the vulnerability of children and the exclusion of disabled and indigenous peoples. It also noted one positive change: enhanced information and communication technology. The conference declaration referred to the concept of health as including mental and spiritual wellbeing. The conference repeated the call from previous international conferences for partnerships, alliances, networks and collaborations to work together to improve health. However, the conference statement regretted that since the adoption of the Ottawa Charter, a significant number of resolutions had been accepted in support of health promotion but had not always been followed by action. It was the first global conference to urge the WHO and its member states to monitor performance through appropriate indicators and targets, and to report on progress at regular intervals.

The Nairobi Conference on Health Promotion (2009)

The outcome of this conference was a *Call to action*, published by the WHO (2009b). The conference attracted over 600 delegates, some participating online, and more than 100 countries were represented. It reaffirmed the values, principles and action strategies of health promotion codified by the Ottawa Charter in

1986 and in subsequent global conferences on health promotion. The document *Call to action* made some impressive claims for health promotion, stating that: 'Health promotion is the most cost-effective strategy to improve health and quality of life and reduces health inequities and poverty' (WHO, 2009b, p 1).

Health promotion also increases people's control over their health and necessary resources for wellbeing. According to the conference's statement, health promotion had demonstrated its effectiveness and return on investment (ROI). The document called on nations to resolve the gap in implementing agreed policies by disseminating compelling evidence on the social, economic, health and other benefits of health promotion to key sectors. As in preceding global conferences on health promotion, the Nairobi *Call to action* (WHO, 2009b) called for continuing individual and community empowerment.

The Helsinki Global Conference on Health Promotion (2013)

This conference published a *Health in all policies* statement calling on nations worldwide to prioritise health and equity as a core responsibility of governments to its peoples. It also urged governments to include communities, social movements and civil society in the development, implementation and monitoring of *Health in all policies*, building health literacy in the population. It stated that such an approach must consider health impacts across all sectors, such as agriculture, education, the environment, housing and transport, to achieve better health outcomes.

The Shanghai Global Conference on Health Promotion (2016)

This conference's pervading theme was sustainable development. It focused on the United Nations' *2030 Agenda for sustainable development* and set out to pursue the '5 Ps' of that agenda:

• **Planet**: Protect the planet for present and future generations; promote sustainable consumption and production; manage natural resources; take action on climate change.

- **People**: Eradicate poverty in all aspects; promote people's potential and dignity; enhance equality in a healthy environment.
- **Prosperity**: Ensure prosperous, comfortable lives for people; ensure economic, social and technological advances in harmony with nature.
- **Peace**: Foster a peaceful, fair and for-all-people society without fear and violence.
- **Partnership**: Mobilise necessary resources; enhance global partnerships; strengthen global solidarity based on the participation of all countries, all target groups and all people. (Adapted from *Transforming our world: the 2030 Agenda for Sustainable Development*, UN General Assembly, ©2015, United Nations. Reprinted with the permission of the United Nations.)

In addition, the conference emphasised the need to strengthen good governance for health through action across all government sectors, to promote health literacy and to create healthy cities in an increasingly urbanised global population.

The WHO

The guidelines for all the aforementioned global conferences on health promotion were laid down in 1977 by the World Health Assembly (WHA), which decided that the main targets of governments and the WHO should be the attainment, by all the people of the world and by the year 2000, of a level of health that would permit them to lead a socially and economically productive life (WHA, 1977). The informing principles of the WHA can be summarised as follows:

- Health is a fundamental human right and a social goal. Policies should be reoriented to focus on maintaining and improving health.
- An equitable distribution of health resources, both within and between countries, should be a fundamental goal.
- Health is shaped by many factors: social, economic, lifestyle and environment. Governments should adopt healthy public

policies that strongly reflect health priorities and that are based on assessments of their health impact.

- Health policies must be pre-emptive and precautionary, the aim being to prevent problems arising at the earliest possible stage.
- Health promotion must include and involve the community while at the same time promoting healthy lifestyles and supportive environments.
- Health services must be reoriented towards primary health care and promoting health rather than simply treating illness.
- Clear performance targets and review mechanisms must be adopted to guide health strategies and achieve their objectives. (Baggott, 2004)

In the same year as the Ottawa Charter on Health Promotion was launched, the WHO published its policy document *Healthy cities* (Davies and Kelly, 1992). Its main objectives were:

- a focus on improving the health of the poor and disadvantaged;
- a need to reorientate medical services and health systems away from hospitals and towards primary care;
- an emphasis on public involvement;
- a need to establish partnerships between the public, private and voluntary sectors.

By 1991, more than 300 cities in the WHO European Region had accepted the principles of *Healthy cities*. In 1999, the European Region set out 21 targets for the 21st century. These consisted of short- and longer-term objectives:

- The targets to be achieved **by 2005** were: all member states to have health research, information and communication systems to support the implementation of *Health for all*, which should engage groups and organisations throughout the public and private sectors and civil society.
  - **By 2010**, there should be better access to primary care; the management of the health sector should be geared towards health outcomes; member states should have sustainable finance; health practitioners should have

acquired appropriate knowledge, attitudes and skills to protect and promote health.

○ **By 2015**, consumption of tobacco, alcohol and psychoactive substances should have been significantly reduced; people should have greater opportunities to live in healthy physical and social environments at home, school and in the local community.

○ **By 2020**, people over 65 years old should have the opportunity to enjoy their full health potential and to play an active social role; people's mental health should be improved with access to comprehensive services; morbidity, disability and premature mortality due to major chronic disease should be reduced to the lowest feasible levels; the health gap between socioeconomic groups within countries should be reduced by at least one fourth. (WHO, 1999)

Setting health targets

Targets to be achieved by a specified date can be expressed either in general terms (such as 'better', 'improved' or 'sustainable') or in precise numbers and percentages. Each technique is subject to potential problems. On the one hand, broad terms are relative, in the sense that they are capable of being interpreted quite differently according to the national context. Different interpretations do not necessarily signify a degree of complacency; for example, accepting that a 5% decrease in tobacco consumption over five years is indicative of a successful health promotion campaign. There may be perfectly justifiable reasons for achieving or falling short of a target, taking into considerations such phenomena as a change of government with different political priorities or an unusually low consumption level as a base for comparison. Apparent failure to meet a specific target expressed in numeral or percentage terms might be the result of an unforeseeable decrease in available funding, or difficulties attracting enough staff to carry out the necessary health promotion interventions.

Health targets on both international and national levels have been revised, often for unexplained reasons,. The original *Health for all* strategy, which set global targets for the year 2000 (WHO,

1981), was altered for the 21st century (WHO, 1998a). In addition, the WHO Regional Office for Europe devised specific *Health for all* targets, which were updated in 1991 and further revised in 1998 (WHO Regional Office, 1998).

In the UK during the 1990s, the government reduced the number of national targets for England. Only four targets were set out in the Green Paper, each of which was intended to be achieved by 2010, using the year 1996 as the baseline. These targets were amended in the subsequent White Paper (Baggott, 2000):

- To reduce the death rate from heart disease, stroke and related illnesses among people under 75 years old by at least two fifths. (The original target was a reduction in the death rate in the under-65s by a third.)
- To reduce the death rate from accidents by at least one fifth and to reduce the rate of serious injury by at least one tenth. (The original target was to reduce accidents by one fifth.)
- To reduce the death rate from cancer among people under 75 by at least one fifth. (The original target was to reduce the death rate in under-65s by one fifth.)
- To reduce the death rate from suicide by at least one fifth. (The original target was a reduction of one sixth.)

Another possible impediment to the achievement of health targets is the absence of any clear direction as to how the targets are to be achieved. This is understandable when discussions in global conferences focus on generally agreed policies and lack the time to set out recommended means of implementing them. However, the question arises as to whether health promotion is the most effective way to challenge and overcome health inequalities and avoidable threats to a population's health. For example, a key statement from the Sunsdvall Conference stressed that the way towards improved health, particularly in countries experiencing extreme poverty and deprivation, lay in making the physical, social, economic and political environment conducive to health. Similarly, the eight fundamental conditions and resources for health detailed in the Ottawa Charter are not in the gift of any health promotion policy or programme –

except, perhaps, as a contribution to education in the form of health education.

A report from the WHO Commission on the social determinants of health (WHO, 2008) drew attention to broad issues that needed to be addressed by governments, and not exclusively by the health sector. Its three principles of action were:

- Improve the conditions of daily life – the circumstances in which people are born, grow, live, work and age.
- Tackle the unequal distribution of power, money and resources – the structural drivers of those conditions of daily life – globally, nationally and locally.
- Measure the problem, evaluate action, expand the knowledge base, develop a workforce that is trained in the social determinants of health and raise public awareness about the social determinants of health.

The Commission's report, *Closing the gap in a generation*, closed by questioning whether the gaps detailed in the second point above can be realised within a generation. It concluded that this was a long-term agenda requiring investment in major changes in social policies, economic arrangements and political action. At the centre of this action should be the empowerment of people, communities and countries that currently do not have their fair share of resources. 'What is needed now is the political will to implement these eminently difficult but feasible changes' (WHO, 2008, p 38).

WHO regions

There are six WHO regions: Africa; the Americas; South East Asia; Europe, the Eastern Mediterranean and the Western Pacific. It is interesting to discover whether each region has similar or different sets of health priorities in the context of health promotion.

African Region

The report by the Regional Director (2016) provides a detailed account of the level and types of diseases that present the health authorities with the greatest challenges and how the challenge is being dealt with. The African Region continues to have a high burden of disease compared with other regions, largely due to a lack of funding. For example, most of the 47 member states lack facilities and trained staff to prevent cervical cancer or detect it at an early stage. Non-communicable diseases (NCDs), disabilities, violence and injuries are an increasing problem. It is projected that by 2025, 55% of all deaths will be the result of NCDs and injuries.

In terms of a crucial component of health promotion – vaccination – there have been important successes. The Ebola virus has been contained and progress is being made in reducing victims of the Zika virus. The region is also continuing to promote immunisation as the most cost-effective lifesaving intervention, especially for children. Strides are also being made in using an oral polio vaccine to prevent the disease occurring and in dealing with other vaccine-preventable illnesses, such as HIV/AIDS, tuberculosis, malaria and neglected tropical diseases. One encouraging outcome is that deaths from HIV/AIDS in the region have decreased by nearly 50% over the past decade, and deaths from malaria by 66% between 2000 and 2015. However, those most likely to die from malaria are children under five years old, and 2.3 million of those suffering from HIV/AIDS are under the age of 15. One disturbing trend has been the very serious outbreak of yellow fever, which started in Angola in 2015, and the continuing problem of sickle cell disease.

Although many diseases prevalent in the African Region do not affect other regions, the Regional Director's report shares with many countries the same concerns over NCDs and their risk factors. These diseases include cancers, lung diseases, diabetes, mental disorders and oral diseases. The WHO has focused on health promotion, risk reduction, prevention, treatment and monitoring of NCDs. The African Region is addressing the main risk factors, which are tobacco use, harmful use of alcohol, physical inactivity and unhealthy diets – the same targets in health promotion initiatives in the UK and many other countries. The report also evidences a keen awareness of the social determinants of health, which are due in part to rapid urbanisation and lifestyle changes. Policies are in place to tackle outbreaks of cholera through cleaner drinking water and improved sanitation. Other risk factors include poverty, food insecurity, environmental degradation, unemployment and gender inequity. To combat these potential threats to health, the report calls for increased investment in health research and development, and health information systems to deliver quality health data for decision-making.

In 2013, a report on health promotion strategy by the African Regional Office summed up the importance of health promotion for sustained health improvement:

> Health promotion interventions are essential in order to effectively address specific public health problems including maternal and child diseases, HIV/AIDS, tuberculosis, malaria, neglected tropical diseases, noncommunicable diseases including malnutrition. The interventions seek to promote healthy behaviours and empower individuals, families, households and communities to take necessary action and to reinforce the desired structural changes through policies, legislation and regulations. (WHO Regional Office for Africa, 2013, p 2)

South East Asia Region

There are 11 countries in the South East Asia Region. The Regional Strategy for Health Promotion (WHO South East Asia Regional Office, 2008) evolved from commitments and actions contained in the Bangkok Charter for Health Promotion (2005). This called for member countries to make health promotion a core responsibility for all government policies and practices, and to ensure health promotion activities are addressed within the existing social, economic, environmental, political and cultural contexts. The regional strategy emphasised the importance of addressing health inequities and the impact of social determinants of health, which have a negative influence on lifestyles and health outcomes for individuals and communities.

The report listed the specific health promotion challenges requiring innovative approaches:

- resource mobilisation and allocation, including the adoption of alternative sources of financing for promoting health;
- addressing complex socioeconomic and cultural changes at family and community levels;
- involving the whole of government (not only health ministries) to address the social determinants of health;
- actively engaging civil society, the private sector and nongovernmental organisations (NGOs) in health promotion;
- strengthening the capacity for health promotion across sectors;
- evidence-gathering regarding the efficacy of health promotion, and the utilisation of such evidence in policy decisions and programming.

The regional strategy also stressed the need for much greater opportunities for training in health promotion at undergraduate and postgraduate levels.

Norton (2016), senior healthcare advisor at PwC South East Asia Consulting, stated in an interview for *Health Care Asia Magazine* that a notable trend in the region was the ageing population, with Singapore and Thailand having the highest percentage of over 65s in the region. Overall, the percentage of people over 65 in the region is expected to more than quadruple by 2050. This will significantly increase the number of women with osteoporosis. Rapid epidemiological transition is also occurring, with the disease burden shifting from infectious to chronic diseases. In Indonesia, NCDs account for 64% of all deaths, and almost 200 million of the world's 370 million people diagnosed with diabetes live in Asia. The South East Asian countries are also experiencing high cancer rates, the most common being lung, breast, liver and colorectal cancers. Haddad et al. (2015) regretted the weak evidence base and very few credible impact assessments of interventions, and referred to a disturbing coexistence of both under- and over-nutrition in the region. They noted that nowhere have overweight rates risen as fast as in the regions of South East Asia and the Pacific. For countries for which data are available, the two regions contain nearly half of individuals worldwide living in an environment in which malnutrition is 'stagnant' and obesity levels are rising.

Americas Region

There are 35 countries in the WHO Americas region. However, they are so diverse that the Pan American Health Organisation has found it problematic to produce health promotion policies that will suit each country. Franceschini and Rice (2011) asserted that trying to decrease inequities in health is one of the biggest challenges facing the countries of the Americas, given the enormous social, economic, political, climatic and ethnic variations in the region, which is still one of the most unequal in terms of wealth and health. The authors carried out 15 case studies, all of which emphasised the centrality of community participation and empowerment for the successful planning, implementation and sustainability of health promotion initiatives and intersectoral collaboration. Despite all the case studies reporting positive outcomes, there was a relative lack of systematic evaluations of health promotion actions. Potvin and McQueen (2008) also agreed on the need for rigorous evaluation of health promotion in their study of evaluation practices in the Americas.

The move to steer away from exclusively clinical interventions towards public health and health promotion became evident in the United States in the 1990s. During this period, according to Speers (1996), the goal of health promotion came to be defined as the absence of disease, with an emphasis on reducing risk factors by changing behaviours. One incentive was the advent of HIV with no medical intervention available to prevent or control the infection. Only health education and health promotion strategies were effective in preventing the spread of disease. The second incentive was the realisation that most deaths in the US are preventable; tobacco, poor diet and physical inactivity accounted for 30% of deaths annually, and sexual behaviour, firearm use, drug and alcohol use, toxic agents and motor vehicles were the other culprits. The main goal of health promotion was creating health for all people by achieving environmental and social equity. For example, poverty, a major cause of ill health, is three times higher among African and Hispanic Americans than among the rest of the population. Various cancers, HIV infection, tuberculosis and diabetes are disproportionately suffered by the poor, as are injuries and infant mortality. In line with the constant plea for valid evidence about the effectiveness of health promotion policies, Speers (1996) made the following observation:

> The methodologies of epidemiology and clinical research cannot be the standard for evaluating health promotion; randomized clinical trials, for example, are of little use in determining whether a health promotion program is effective. Qualitative methodologies, including new research paradigms such as participatory research, are much more likely to elucidate the relationship between health promotion interventions and outcomes. (p 70)

The US Centers for Disease Control and Prevention's (2014) National Prevention Strategy 'helps move the nation away from a health care system focused on sickness and disease to one focused on wellness and prevention' (p 1). The strategy laid down four key policy areas – healthy and safe community environments; clinical and community preventative services; empowered people; elimination of health disparities – and seven priority areas:

- tobacco-free living;
- preventing drug abuse and excessive alcohol use;
- healthy eating;
- active living;
- injury- and violence-free living;
- reproductive and sexual health;
- mental and emotional wellbeing.

For Latin America, the World Economic Forum (2016) listed five challenges:

- **Access to health services:** Approximately 30% of the population of Latin America and the Caribbean do not have access to healthcare for economic reasons.
- **Epidemiologic transition and NCDs:** During the previous century, the region experienced health issues seen in many developing countries, with high levels of infectious and acute diseases placing pressure on weak health systems.
- **Training and distribution of human resources in health:** Few countries in the region meet international indicators, such as number of doctors/nurses per 10,000 inhabitants or hospital beds per 1,000 inhabitants.
- **Inequalities in health:** Latin America has a high level of inequity and inequality. Many sections of the population are at a higher risk, as health problems are often influenced by societal factors such as education, income and ethnicity.
- **Financing health systems:** Changes in patterns of disease and rising ageing populations increase the cost of healthcare. This system becomes unsustainable because it encourages a system based on disease and not health.

The measures needed to meet and overcome these challenges are as follows:

- The health of a population is the result of decisions taken at the political, economic and social levels. Therefore, health problems should be solved by interdisciplinary and intersector action, and not only by health professionals.
- There must be increased investment in public health that encourages prevention instead of funding based on illness. This involves health promotion and disease prevention.
- Health problems such as chronic NCDs must be addressed by improving primary healthcare and promoting healthy lifestyles.
- Technology and interaction between the public and private sectors can provide solutions to the problems of access to health services.

Eastern Mediterranean Region

There are 21 countries in the Eastern Mediterranean Region. The *Strategy for Health Promotion* (WHO, 2008) in the region included most of the key policies that feature in the other regions' strategic documents:

- the need to acknowledge the social determinants of health;
- a multisectoral response to minimising the negative impact on health of poverty;
- a campaign to improve unhealthy lifestyles;
- the requirement of increased financing for health promotion.

The document urged all countries in the region to be more proactive in dealing with emerging risk factors (for example, sedentary lifestyles, unhealthy diet, smoking and drug abuse) and with the health consequences of rates of obesity, diabetes, injuries, cancer and cardiovascular disease. Not surprisingly, in this region the problem of alcohol abuse does not arise. One of the most important messages in the report is that health promotion is cost-effective; it improves health and has a positive impact on economic development through gains in healthy life years, increased productivity and a decreased economic burden of disease. In particular, ministries of health need to strengthen their role by providing a supportive environment for health promotion activities. The strategy document identified some of the most important challenges for health promotion in the region:

- scarcity of data through which to identify priority problems and evaluate health promotion interventions;
- low priority placed on prevention and promotion from decision-makers and other stakeholders;
- rapid social changes representing a threat to regional cultural characteristics traditionally thought to be protective against ill health or risky health behaviour;
- insufficient legislation or non-enforcement of existing laws on health promotion;
- inadequate resources (both human and financial) for health promotion interventions and activities;

- limited intersectoral cooperation and coordination;
- inadequate involvement of the private sector in health promotion.

However, increasing conflict in the region is threatening to undermine any progress that has been made in improving health and life expectancy. A report by the Institute for Health Metrics and Evaluation (IHME) (2017) confirmed that improvements in the past 20 years are being subverted by wars and civil unrest. Conflicts have destroyed infrastructures in several nations, and with inadequate water and sanitation systems in some countries there is a pressing need to ensure outbreaks and illnesses are properly controlled. Moreover, many physicians and health professionals are fleeing their home countries in search of stability and safety. In addition, conflicts in the region have displaced millions of people. Outbreaks of infectious diseases in camps with poor sanitation and lack of immunisation facilities worsen the health of refugees and pose major obstacles to health efforts. Frequent attacks on vaccination teams have greatly slowed immunisation campaigns, and polio has again become a major concern, especially in refugee camps, at a time when the region was close to eradicating it.

Chronic diseases such as ischaemic heart disease and diabetes cause a greater burden to health in the region than communicable diseases such as diarrhoea and tuberculosis. Childhood malnutrition is the leading health risk in low-income countries such as Somalia, Afghanistan and Yemen. Between 1990 and 2013, life expectancy in the region increased from 65 to 71, which is a sign of general progress, with Qatar having the highest life expectancy (81 for men and 83 for women). Across the region, mental health and drug-use disorders have increased significantly since 1990. These disorders caused 7.3% of premature deaths and illness between 1990 and 2008, nearly doubling from 3.9% in 1990. The IHME study reported that this rise has not been met with investment in prevention by most countries. The region is also recording a worrying upward trend in the incidence of traffic injuries. External factors, including increased temperatures and droughts causing water shortages, are a major threat to health in many Eastern Mediterranean countries.

European Region

There are 53 countries in the European Region. In 2010, a report by the Regional Office identified a number of concerns shared by the other regions: people are increasingly mobile, the population is ageing, socioeconomic inequities are growing within and between countries and countries were seriously affected by the global financial crisis of 2010. Moreover, the region was experiencing an epidemic of NCDs, including cardiovascular diseases, cancer and mental disorders. In addition, communicable diseases – polio, tuberculosis (TB), HIV/AIDS and influenza – comprised a major health challenge. Environmental factors such as climate change, air and water quality and the use of chemicals were causing new risks to health, such as respiratory and waterborne diseases.

The correlation between poor health and socioeconomic disadvantage is clear. For example, the infant mortality rate in the poorest countries in the region is 25 times that in the richest. The report also recognised that the social determinants of health – poverty; education; employment; housing; social exclusion and control over one's own life – needed to be tackled. As in other regions, the European report emphasised intersectoral collaboration as crucial to the success of disease prevention and health promotion policies and interventions. It also targeted unhealthy lifestyles that contributed significantly to poor health.

A more recent report from the Regional Office (CHRODIS, 2015) analysed the situation in 14 European countries. It found that 'while much is being done across Europe, there remains an urgent need to increase investment in health promotion and disease prevention' (p 28). It added that there are clear differences in levels and sources of funding and capacity across the partner countries in relation to health promotion and primary prevention systems and structures.

Because public health budgets are constrained and only a very small percentage of health expenditures are allocated to prevention and health promotion, this financing strategy needs to be reconsidered, as investment in health promotion has been shown to be cost-effective. Member states need to share the many examples of good practice highlighted in the report.

Western Pacific Region

There are 27 countries in this region. The problem of the persistent levels of NCDs mirrors the situation throughout all the WHO regions. However, the Western Pacific Region is the only one to have developed a distinct Mental Health Action Plan (WHO, 2013). This comprehensive report has an all-encompassing goal: to promote mental wellbeing; prevent mental disorders; provide care; enhance recovery; promote human rights and reduce mortality, morbidity and disability for persons with mental disorders. It states that this will require a multisectoral approach with an emphasis on early intervention, since many mental health problems are manifest before the age of 14. The action plan has as its core the globally accepted principle that there is 'no health without mental health' (p 8).

The term 'mental disorders' used in the action plan includes conditions that cause a high burden of illness, such as depression; bipolar disorder; schizophrenia; anxiety disorder; dementia; substance misuse; intellectual disabilities and development and behavioural disorders with onset usually occurring in childhood and adolescence, including autism. For dementia and substance misuse, additional prevention strategies may be required; for example, to reduce the harmful use of alcohol. The plan also deals with the prevention of suicide. It acknowledges that certain individuals and groups may be at significantly higher risk of experiencing mental health problems, which may (but do not necessarily) include people living in poverty; people with chronic health conditions; children exposed to maltreatment and neglect; adolescents exposed to substance misuse; lesbian, gay, bisexual and transgender persons; prisoners, and people exposed to conflict, natural disasters or other emergencies. Domestic violence, unemployment and stress are also potential causes of mental ill health.

In addition, according to the action plan, there is evidence that depression predisposes people to myocardial infarction and diabetes – both of which increase the likelihood of depression. The economic consequences of these health issues are also considerable in terms of lost economic output. Because of stigmatisation and discrimination, persons with mental disorders often have their human rights violated, with restrictions on the right to work and education. The Western Pacific Action Plan calls for the need for evidence-based practice, for many more professionals able to deal with mental health problems, for increased funding and for the involvement of people with mental disorders in mental health advocacy; policy; planning; legislation; service provision; monitoring, research and evaluation. Health-promoting schools can also play a part in fostering good physical and mental health.

Apart from this special attention to the needs of persons experiencing mental health problems, the Western Pacific Region reflects the global issue of risks involved with unhealthy lifestyles – lack of physical activity, poor diet, use of tobacco and abuse of alcohol – all of which can contribute to overweight and obesity, raised blood pressure and high cholesterol levels.

The World Health Organization

The WHO Statistics (2017) set down six lines of action for member states to follow:

- intersectoral action by multiple stakeholders;
- health systems strengthened by universal health coverage;
- respect for equity and human rights;
- sustainable funding;
- scientific research and innovation;
- monitoring and evaluation.

With regard to the first item in the list, the report points out that there are many opportunities for improving health through intersectoral action. These are set out in Table 7.1.

Table 7.1: Opportunities for improving health through intersectoral action

Exposure	Key health outcomes	Intersectoral action
Inadequate water and hygiene	Diarrhoeal disease, malnutrition, hepatitis, typhoid, poliomyelitis	Action by water, sanitation and education sectors
Poverty and food insecurity	Deaths of children under 5	Social welfare programmes for better child nutrition
Air pollution	Cardiovascular diseases, chronic obstructive pulmonary disease, respiratory infections, lung cancer	Health-promoting urban design and transport systems
Substandard and unsafe housing and unsafe communities	Asthma, CVDs, injuries, violent deaths	Implementation of housing standards and urban designs that promote health
Hazardous, unsafe and unhealthy work environments	COPD, CVD, lung cancer, leukaemia, hearing loss, back pain, injuries, depression	Labour sector promotion of occupational standards and workers' rights
Exposure to carcinogens through unsafe chemicals and foods	Cancers, neurological disorders	Sound management of chemicals and food across the food industry and agriculture sector
Unhealthy food consumption and lack of physical activity	Obesity, CVDs, diabetes, cancers, dental caries	Improving product standards and public spaces
Inadequate childcare and learning environments	Suboptimal cognitive, social and physical development	Early child development programmes and improved female education

Source: WHO (2017)

The WHO report (2017) stresses the need to measure outcomes in the following areas:

- reproductive, maternal, newborn and child health;
- infectious diseases;
- NCDs and mental health;
- injuries and violence;
- environmental risks;
- health risks and disease outbreaks.

Under the first five of these headings, the report provides statistics based on the data available in 2015:

- **Global maternal mortality rate**: 216 per 100,000 live births. Target: to reduce this rate to fewer than 79 by 2030.
- **Malaria cases**: 212 million, a decrease of 41% since 2000. The worst incidence is in the African Region, where children under 5 account for 70% of all deaths. TB remains a global health problem; there were 1.4 million deaths, the highest rate being in the African Region.
- **Deaths from NCDs**: 40 million, primarily through cardiovascular disease, cancer, chronic respiratory disease and diabetes.
- **Deaths from traffic injuries**: 1.25 million, an increase of 13% since 2000, with the most vulnerable being in the 15–29 age group.
- **Unsafe water and sanitation**: 92% of the world's population are living in places where WHO air quality standards are not being met.

The report then listed targets to be reached by the year 2030:

- to reduce the global maternal mortality ratio to less than 70 per 100,000 live births;
- to end preventable deaths of newborns and children under 5 years of age, and reduce neonatal mortality to a maximum of 12 for 1,000 live births and under-5 mortality to a maximum of 25 per 1,000 live births;

- to end the epidemics of AIDS, TB, malaria and neglected tropical diseases and communicable disease;
- to reduce by one third premature mortality from NCDs through prevention and treatment, and to promote mental health and wellbeing;
- to strengthen the prevention and treatment of substance abuse, including narcotic drug abuse and harmful use of alcohol;
- by 2020, to halve the number of global deaths and injuries from road traffic accidents.

It also provided statistics on life expectancy in all the WHO regions, shown below.

WHO region	Life expectancy
African	60
Americas	77
South East Asia	68.9
Europe	76.8
Eastern Mediterranean	68.8
West Pacific	76.6

Equality and equity

The Global Conference and reports from the WHO regional offices refer to the need to counter the problems of health **inequalities** and health **inequities**. These need to be clearly distinguished from each other to guard against possible confusion. Laverack (2014) places the term inequity in the context of **social injustice**, which reflects differences in wealth and power. Efforts to reduce inequities involve changing the unfair distribution of social and material resources. Governments can have a significant impact on the social determinants of health through the policies and legislation they authorise. Laverack (2014) goes on to list some actions that governments can take, which Wilkinson (2003) proposed. These are:

- improving the teaching and resource allocation to schools;
- ensuring a minimum wage and regulated working hours;
- creating better opportunities to find work;
- protecting vulnerable and marginalised groups;
- providing preventative services and parental education about childcare;
- creating better access to affordable childcare facilities;
- building community support and social interaction;
- improving access to public transport;
- improving access to public exercise facilities, such as cycle paths.

However, Laverack (2014) states: 'A health inequity is a difference (an inequality) in health that is significant in the number of people affected ... The inequalities in everyday living include unequal access to health care and education, conditions of work and the limited opportunities to lead a healthy life' (p 69). Elsewhere, Laverack (2014) advocates sustainable programmes that aim to build healthy public policy and supportive environments for health in ways that 'improve living conditions, support healthy lifestyles and achieve greater equity in health' (p 44). Unfortunately, the expression 'equity in health' blurs the distinction between the concepts of health inequality and health inequity. Indeed, it would probably be preferable to use the term 'equity' without the preceding word 'health'. Gottwald and Goodman-Brown (2012) refer to 'health inequity' as a situation relating to different opportunities for health; for example, as a result of access to resources such as nutritious food, housing or health services. Health inequalities are differences in the health status between individuals, groups or populations, which may be the result of health inequities.

Baggott (2000) makes the point that the concepts 'equality' and 'equity' are often used interchangeably even though they have different meanings. Inequality, he argues, is neither good nor bad; it depends on the circumstances. For example, the fact that younger people tend to enjoy better health than elderly people is not regarded as inequitable. In contrast, the poorer health of lower-income people relative to the more affluent is viewed by many as inequitable. Concepts of equity and inequity are therefore rooted in beliefs about 'what should be' (p 221). There have been a number of contributors to the discussion of what constitutes 'equity' in the field of health policy (Sen 1985; LeGrand, 1987; Whitehead, 1992; Pereira, 1993; Drever and Whitehead, 1997). In essence, this distinction should suffice: equity refers to the *nature of a situation*, which is perceived to be fair or just or the opposite. It has an intrinsically ethical dimension. In the context of health, this usually refers to the opportunity to gain access to the means by which one can enjoy a standard of health comparable to the healthiest sections of society. Health equality, or its opposite, represents the *outcome* of an equitable or inequitable situation. The outcome may be a lower or comparable standard of health, but whether this outcome is construed as acceptable or otherwise depends on the nature of the situation. In Baggott's example, the situation of being young rather than elderly is certainly outside the control of the individual, but this cannot be interpreted as unjust.

Concluding thoughts

Across the globe, in all six WHO regions, there is substantial agreement on both the main health problems and the means of combating them. Great emphasis is placed on acknowledging the social and economic determinants of health and the effect that increased urbanisation is having on the health of populations. There is also a shared commitment to a strategy based on intersectoral collaboration, which distracts from positioning clinical interventions as the sole means of improving a nation's health. There is, however, an apparent contradiction in asserting that health promotion has a proven track record in preventing diseases and providing a cost-effective approach to health issues, and in the same statement calling for much more extensive and rigorous evaluation of health promotion interventions. On the face of it, the Nairobi Conference declaration that health promotion reduces health inequities and poverty demands convincing supporting evidence. Here again, the term 'inequities' is probably more aptly termed 'inequalities'.

Ever since the setting of targets became integral to global health policies, there has been no explanation as to why the targets have not been met. This is unfortunate, because such information could be extremely useful in helping to redesign policies and reallocate resources to remedy the identified defects or prevailing factors. Heed could be taken of the Bangkok Conference recommendation that regions should use performance indicators to monitor progress towards achieving agreed outcomes. Such a lack of evidence is relevant to any discussion of the future of health promotion.

EIGHT

The future for health promotion

Civil society organisations

Some of the most flourishing health promotion initiatives are run by organisations within 'civil society'. For example, village halls throughout the UK hold classes dedicated to maintaining and improving people's health. These might include pilates, yoga, dance, tai chi and Zumba (a system of exercises performed to Latin American and other forms of music). Badminton and tennis clubs meet in schools and other community venues. Local football, rugby and hockey clubs abound, and local authorities (LAs) provide leisure centres where residents can participate in a range of physical pursuits such as swimming, weight training and fitness. While a token attendance or membership fee is usually payable to take part in such activities, these are not-for-profit organisations. Outside these community enterprises are commercial ventures that nevertheless contribute to health promotion, such as gyms, golf clubs and slimming ventures, although their membership fees might preclude those on low incomes from joining.

In addition, as representatives of civil society, many charities have one or more of the three potential components of health promotion strategies as their primary aim. For example, as noted in Chapter Six, mental health charities mostly help people to cope with their condition and to progress towards a release from suffering without resorting to clinical treatments. Third-sector organisations are also active in supporting drug and alcohol abusers towards rehabilitation, while numerous charities focus on fundraising activities to finance research or practical assistance for people afflicted with specific physical diseases, such as cancer, multiple sclerosis, heart conditions and diabetes. These organisations bear witness to the oft-quoted assertion that health promotion relies on a multisectoral approach, which in effect is a combination – if not necessarily a partnership – between government, business and civil society.

Homelessness

UK health survey reports make scant reference to the health and health needs of homeless persons. Although discussion of the health impact of people living in 'poverty' features in reports, scholarly articles and books on health promotion, homeless people are not mentioned. However, those third-sector organisations that raise funds to help support homeless people – such as The Big Issue, Joseph Rowntree Foundation and HomelessLink – clearly recognise the relatively poor health conditions of people sleeping rough, living temporarily in homeless shelters or 'sofa surfing'. The Salvation Army is also active in catering for the health needs of homeless persons, while Centrepoint helps young homeless persons (aged 16–25) to find homes and jobs.

In England, HomelessLink reported that 86% of homeless persons claimed to have some form of mental illness, 44% had been diagnosed with a mental health issue, 41% said they had taken drugs or were recovering from a drug problem and 27% said they were recovering from an alcohol problem (HomelessLink, 2017). All of these health problems would be an appropriate target for health promotion interventions within a public health policy. As Frankish et al. (2005) have stated, homelessness has a direct adverse impact on physical health, while certain health conditions – particularly mental illness – can contribute to, and then be exacerbated by, homelessness. There is also evidence that the mortality rate among homeless persons is higher than the rest of the population.

Power et al. (1999) argue that 'there have been extensive reviews of homelessness and health, along with calls for urgent action, but little attention has been paid to the health promotion needs of homeless people, and there is no firm evidence base for practice' (p 590). Their article merits extensive coverage, since it remains of contemporary relevance and importance. They specify the challenge to health promotion policies and the potential means of providing appropriate interventions:

One challenge for health promotion is to develop and deliver appropriate initiatives to a heterogeneous population that is not easy to categorise but has a wide range of needs. The healthcare priorities of a young man sleeping on the streets differ from those of a single mother in temporary accommodation. To be homeless means more than just the absence of secure accommodation. Homelessness has as much to do with social exclusion as with bricks and mortar, and demands a range of health promotion strategies. (p 590)

The authors list a number of barriers to health promotion among homeless people:

- Workers with homeless people are often isolated. There is little coordination or collaboration between health promotion agencies.
- Health promotion departments rarely set up initiatives specifically targeting homelessness and housing.
- Homeless people can feel alienated from health promotion materials, which often require high levels of literacy.
- Although homeless people are concerned about health-related problems, low self-esteem and low expectations prevent them from engaging with health promotion activities.

They conclude by first recommending that homeless people be involved in formative evaluations to identify the best venues and means of delivering health promotion; and second by arguing that the variety of health needs among homeless people provides an opportunity for intersectoral health promotion activities. Coles et al. (2012) echo the first recommendation, maintaining that in order to achieve success, health improvement interventions must incorporate and be tailored to the lifestyle and individual needs of homeless persons. The health promotion approach must be participative and client-centred.

It is perhaps timely for health promotion organisations and health service practitioners to reflect and agree upon a very positive strategy to help improve the physical and mental health needs of homeless people. The Homelessness Reduction Act was passed in the UK parliament in 2017, and is due to be implemented in 2018. The Act will impose a new duty on LAs to prevent the homelessness of all families and single people, regardless of priority need. The intention is to support people to either stay in their accommodation or find somewhere permanent to live.

Then and now

Just as homelessness was a significant social problem in Victorian Britain and earlier times, public health issues of the past have either re-emerged in 21st-century Britain or were never removed. Chapter Two detailed how governments in previous centuries reacted to widespread diseases that claimed the lives of thousands of citizens in various parts of the UK. Two of the more persistent causes of ill health were air pollution (known as 'miasma') and the pollution of rivers, in particular the Thames. In 2017, these pernicious phenomena have returned.

Air pollution

Levels of nitrogen dioxide, emitted mainly by diesel cars, have been above legal limits in almost 90% of urban areas in the UK since 2010; in 2016, parliament declared this problem to be a public health emergency (Carrington, 2017). One possible solution was the scrapping of diesel cars and giving a financial incentive to diesel car owners to replace their vehicles with petrol-fuelled or electric-powered vehicles (Mason, 2017). Air pollution in the UK is thought to cause up to 40,000 deaths a year, seriously affecting people suffering from asthma. However, environmentalists have described the UK government's policy, declared in May 2017, as 'weak' and 'woefully inadequate' (Carrington, 2017). The policy looks to LAs to take the necessary steps to reduce air pollution in their areas, possibly by creating clean air zones. Transport campaigners want the government to take measures similar to those in Germany and France, where car makers are forced to pay for upgrades to their vehicles to cut levels of air pollution.

A World Health Organization (WHO, 2017) report has highlighted the seriousness of the situation in the UK, where indoor and outdoor pollution is responsible for 25.7 deaths per 100,000 – worse than 14 other European countries, and worse than Mexico, Brazil and Argentina. In the US, the death rate per 100,000 is 12.1. The problem of air pollution re-emerged dramatically during what is known as the Great Smog of 1952 in London. The Clean Air Act 1956 followed, and was replaced by the Clean Air Act 1993. This Act made it an offence for any householder to allow smoke emissions from a chimney unless the smoke was caused by an authorised fireplace and fuel. Today, the Department of the Environment, Food and Rural Affairs is responsible for monitoring levels of air pollution and other environmental hazards.

River pollution

As noted in Chapter Two, the increased population and urbanisation as a result of the burgeoning Industrial Revolution in Britain brought sanitation problems and poor housing. These conditions were not confined to London. In 1840, the River Aire in Leeds was infested with 'refuse from water closets, cesspools, privies, common drains, dung-hill drainings, infirmary refuse, wastes from slaughter-houses, chemical soap, gas ... pig manure, old urine wash ... dead animals and occasionally a decomposed human body' (Wohl, 1984, p 235). The likelihood of a similar environmental disaster happening in the 21st century seems unthinkable. Yet in 2017, Thames Water was fined an unprecedented £20 million for allowing 1.4 billion litres of raw polluted sewage and a variety of sanitary products to be jetted into the River Thames and countryside rivers in three English counties. The company had been fined £1 million for river pollution in 2016. The Environment Agency brought the prosecution. Between 2014 and 2016, four other water companies had been fined for similar breaches of quality standards (*The Independent*, 2014). Instances such as these have not been confined to England. In June 2017, waste from an anaerobic digestion plant contaminated the River Teifi near Lampeter in west Wales (BBC Wales, 2017). In Scotland, 20 rivers have been polluted by toxic chemicals in the past three years (*The Herald*, 2014), and in Northern Ireland the NI Water Company was fined £13,000 in 2016 for polluting a river in County Down (*The Irish News*, 2016).

Health protection

Today in the UK, there are a number of agencies and government departments whose remit is to protect the public from potentially harmful products or natural occurrences that present a threat to public health. From time to time, as with air and river pollution, incidents occur that have to be controlled or remedied, or where legal action is taken against the offenders. The most prominent body in England is the Environment Agency, which has its counterparts in Scotland (the Scottish Environment Protection Agency), Wales (Natural Resources Wales) and Northern Ireland (the Northern Ireland Environment Agency). These share the same functions, which include:

- regulating major industry and waste
- protection against flooding
- monitoring water quality
- treatment of contaminated land
- measures to respond to climate change
- ensuring standards of recycling are maintained
- commercial fisheries: protecting fish stocks; checking river levels
- radioactive substances: issuing and varying permits for radioactive substance sites
- conservation and heritage sites: natural and wildlife conservation; cultural and heritage site conservation
- noise nuisance: issuing environmental permits as part of noise pollution control

Environmental health officers (EHOs) monitor and inspect premises to ensure the public is protected against a number of potential health hazards. Their predecessors were the officers of health and inspectors of nuisances, appointed by the General Board of Health and local boards of health as a result of the

1848 Public Health Act (Lumley, 1859). EHOs are mainly employed by LAs, but they may also work within the NHS, armed services or the government's Food Standards Agency. Their duties are wide-ranging, and include monitoring and inspecting the following:

- food safety
- environmental protection
- noise, radiation and pollution control
- water standards
- health and safety at work
- animal welfare
- waste management
- housing standards

In Wales and Northern Ireland, under their Food Hygiene Ratings Act (in Wales since 2013 and Northern Ireland in 2016), it is mandatory for restaurants, pubs, cafes, takeaways, hotels, supermarkets and other food shops to display their food hygiene rating, ranked from zero to five. In England and Scotland, displaying the rating is voluntary. The inspections check how hygienically the food is handled (how it is prepared, cooked, reheated, cooled and stored), the condition of the structure of the buildings (cleanliness, layout, lighting and ventilation) and how the business manages and records what it does to make sure food is safe. If the rating is under five, the inspecting officer will advise the owners what steps are needed to improve it. If the rating is zero, the food outlet will need to take urgent measures; if those measures do not bring about an improvement, the LA could close down the premises.

Another function EHOs perform under the rubric 'health protection' relates to **health and safety at work**. The Act of 1974 established the Health and Safety Commission (HSC) and the Health and Safety Executive (HSE) in 1975. The first factory inspectors were appointed under the provisions of the Factories Act of 1833. The Mines and Collieries Act followed in 1842. Initially, just four inspectors were responsible for 3,000 textile mills. By 1868, this number had increased to 35.

Today, the HSE is responsible for regulating workplaces employing the majority of the working population, while LA EHOs inspect health and safety conditions in offices, shops and smaller workshops (Baggott, 2000). In 2008, the HSC and HSE merged as the HSE. Legislation from 1833 onwards has played an important role in safeguarding employees from accidents, injuries and exposure to toxic substances – most notably, in the past few decades, exposure to asbestos. In 2010, Lord Young presented his report *Common sense, common safety* ('the Young report') which was a response to the government's concern about public disillusionment with applying the legislation to certain spheres of activity, such as schools and LAs. In a foreword to the report, then Prime Minister David Cameron explained the reasons for the review of current legislation:

> Good health and safety is vitally important. But all too often good, straightforward legislation designed to protect people from major hazards has been extended inappropriately to cover every walk of life, no matter how low risk. As a result, instead of being valued, the standing of health and safety in the eyes of the public has never been lower … A damaging compensation has arisen, as if people can absolve themselves from any personal responsibility for their own actions, with the prospect of lawyers only too willing to pounce with a claim for damages on the slightest pretext. (Young Report, 2010, Foreword)

Apart from recommendations to challenge what the Prime Minister termed 'compensation culture', Lord Young ridiculed some of the more extreme examples of practices carried out in the name of health and safety. One involved a restaurant not issuing toothpicks to customers in case of injury; in another, a teacher warned pupils not to walk under a horse chestnut tree without wearing helmets to ward off falling conkers. LAs that banned certain events on the grounds of health and safety were made to publicise their reasons in detail.

One offshoot of legislation that has not attracted government attention has been the introduction of high-vis clothing in almost every walk of life in which people appear outdoors. While this is a sensible precaution against accidents for those working in potentially dangerous locations (such as railway lines, roads and building sites), as well as for cyclists, the media have been united in their criticism of what is perceived as a totally unnecessary gesture to health and safety. *The Daily Mail*, *The Sunday Times* and *The Telegraph* all railed against the proliferation of **Hi-Vis** attire in every corner of Britain. Their comments were represented in a contribution to BBC News by Jon Kelly (2011): 'To critics, it symbolises everything that is wrong about mollycoddled, risk-averse, health-and-safety-obsessed modern Britain. Hi Vis has come to lend its wearers the mantle of officialdom, licensed to give orders by virtue of their outerwear'.

As well as health problems caused by exhaust emissions, cars have come in for criticism mainly because of the accidents caused by their drivers. Drink-driving laws, speed limits, traffic-calming measures and penalties for using a mobile phone while driving are all intended to reduce avoidable accidents. Perhaps the most contentious issue has been legislation relating to **the wearing of seat belts**. Attempts were made from the 1970s onwards in Britain to introduce a law that would make wearing seat belts mandatory. Even though this had been compulsory in Sweden since 1958, opposition in the UK adopted the same attitude that other health protection policies had stimulated in the 19th century. As noted in Chapter Two, Longmate (1966) recorded a negative reaction in newspapers to the proposed vaccination programme against smallpox and other diseases. The complaint centred on taking a chance rather than being bullied into health. This argument is central to public reaction to government proposals that are intended to protect people against possible damage to their health. Many would prefer to 'take a chance' – to accept the risk, rather than be subjected to a mandatory intervention.

Such was the situation in the face of the 'threat' of seat-belt legislation. The RAC was sceptical, but accepted that a voluntary approach would be acceptable. The police objected because it would be very difficult to enforce, and the Ministry of Transport believed it would be an unwarrantable infringement of civil liberties (National Archives, 2017). In addition, it was argued at the time (the 1960s) that certain individuals – such as 'dwarfs'; 'children'; 'pregnant women'; 'the deformed'; 'seriously obese people'; 'very tall people'; and 'elderly persons' – ought to be exempt if a law was brought in (National Archives, 2017). One of the most strenuous objectors was John Adams, a professor of geography at University College, London. His contention was that the compulsion to wear seat belts would not reduce accidents, but that it would spur drivers to drive at greater speeds, resulting in more rather than fewer road accidents (Adams, 2006). Adams was still arguing his case 20 years after the law was introduced, and later called for the law to be repealed, disputing the figures from the Road Safety Observatory on the number of lives saved and serious injuries avoided due to drivers and passengers wearing seat belts (ROSPA, 2017). In principle, this legislation, he contended, was an unwarranted use of state power and infringed individual liberty. People take risks, so why not have laws banning rock climbing, cycling, drinking alcohol, smoking and eating too many cream buns (Cowley, 2009)?

Today, the only exceptions to the mandatory wearing of seat belts are on medical grounds (which have to be proved by means of a doctor's certificate), a driver reversing or supervising a learner driver who is reversing, a licensed taxi driver and the driver of a goods vehicle that is delivering and travelling no more than 50 metres between stops. Children under the age of 13 must wear a child restraint; children aged 14 years and above must wear a seat belt.

Risks and health promotion

Although the concept of **protection** is not stated as central to the policy of health promotion, it is relevant to certain health promotion objectives and activities. In drawing the public's attention to avoiding certain unhealthy behaviours – such as poor diet, smoking, drinking too much alcohol and not taking enough exercise –health education attempts to protect people from the likelihood of contracting certain illnesses, and even from premature death. Arguably, some people choose not to heed advice along these lines for one or more of the following reasons:

1 They are willing to take the risk because of the satisfaction they derive from leading their particular lifestyle.
2 They object to the government advising them to eat five (or even ten) helpings of fruit and vegetable every day. This is a symptom of the nanny state.
3 They cannot afford to lead a healthier lifestyle even if they wanted to.
4 They are unlikely to be healthy because of circumstances outside their control, such as poor housing, overcrowding or air pollution.

Commentators who subscribe to the social determinants of health position would accept items 3 and 4 on the list as the dominant factors. Another view would be that since people have the responsibility to live a healthy life, they are being irresponsible if they ignore health warnings such as 'SMOKING KILLS' on packets of cigarettes. One key motive among health promotion advocates is to instil a degree of what they would term **health literacy** among the population. To assume that members of the public are unaware of what are healthy and unhealthy lifestyle choices carries with it the possible accusation of being patronising and unhelpful. The media, in whatever format, are awash with articles and messages about how to live a healthy life. With the exception of parents who do not discourage their children from becoming seriously obese, it could be argued that government agencies such as public health trusts should not attempt to interfere in people's lives, however noble their motives (Naidoo and Wills, 2016).

One notable motive that informs health promotion policy is to empower individuals and communities. This strategy has been discussed in previous chapters in terms of what it hopes to achieve. Nevertheless, it has a bearing on the four aforementioned possible explanations for people's noncompliance with authoritative risk warnings. Nutbeam (2000) regarded health literacy as not only imparting information and ensuring people could read pamphlets and make appointments but also as critical to empowerment. However, Laverack (2014) questions whether a health literacy approach in health promotion, which is intended to achieve behaviour change, is consistent and compatible with an empowerment approach. He cites Tengland (2013), who asserts that the behaviour change approach has several ethical problems, several of which have been alluded to in previous chapters. These are that efforts to alter people's behaviour towards a healthier lifestyle are overly paternalistic and often disregard the individual's own perception of what is important. Such efforts can lead to 'victim blaming' and to increased inequalities in health, because they ignore the social determinants of health. While favouring the empowerment approach, Laverack (2014) concedes that it can lead to empowering some groups rather than others. In addition, the focus might not be primarily on health, and empowered people might still choose to behave in ways that risk damaging their health.

A final word on empowerment

It is important to revisit the issue of individual and community empowerment here to explore the validity of its proponents' claims that empowerment should be a central aim of health promotion, now and in the future. One of the frustrations in reading the large corpus of articles on empowerment and health is the somewhat bland acceptance that health promotion's aim to empower individuals and communities is to be commended and encouraged, without identifying what empowerment actually entails.

Woodall et al. (2010) reviewed the relevant literature and found that: 'There is much confusion about what empowerment is and what it means' (p 9). The authors distinguish between individual and community empowerment. The former, they state, means people feeling – and actually having – a sense of control over their lives. This sense of control is important because it has a direct effect on improving an individual's mental and physical health (Wallerstein, 1992; Rissel, 1994; Koelen and Lindstrom, 2005). Woodall et al. (2010) note that **individual empowerment** is limited because it does not consider wider environmental influences on people's health, such as poverty and employment. The solution lies in **community empowerment**. This involves the development of groups of people who take political and social action to create social change through the redistribution of resources and power (Wallerstein, 2002). However, in assessing the health promotion evidence base, Woodall et al. (2010) make the familiar pronouncement that 'although the term empowerment is frequently used, the availability of high-quality research which demonstrates its success for improving individual health and well-being is fairly minimal' (p 13). They then list five examples of evidence indicating that empowerment has resulted in health-related outcomes:

1 Improved self-efficacy and esteem (where 'self-efficacy' is described as 'people's belief about performing a given activity', p 9);
2 Increased knowledge and awareness;
3 Behaviour change;
4 A greater sense of community;
5 A greater sense of control.

In response to these outcomes, one might ask the following questions:

1 What bearing has 'belief' on an individual's actions?
2 Knowledge and awareness of what, and to what end?
3 Behaviour change in what way?
4 In what respects does a greater sense of community impact on a person's health?
5 Greater sense of control over what?

Unfortunately, all five examples of success relate to case studies outside the UK – namely Nepal, Vietnam, Florida and China. This raises further questions about the transferability of evidence to a different social, cultural and political milieu, such as the UK.

Woodall et al.'s (2010) literature review examines the meaning and success of *community empowerment*. They begin by stating that: 'Measuring the impact of empowerment on a community level is very difficult' (2010, p 17). They found few instances where empowerment approaches had made a difference to the actual health and wellbeing of communities. Again, they found that 'where evidence on community empowerment is available, it predominantly comes from outside of the UK and is based mainly in developing countries. The evidence suggests that programmes often find it challenging to quantify the actual differences they make to the health of individuals and communities' (p 21). Gibbon (2000) further undermines the whole strategy of community empowerment, warning that empowerment strategies – for example, involvement in a group – can raise expectations regarding improved health and wellbeing, with the consequence of a feeling of frustration (Gibbon, 2000).

The one UK case study included in the review was the Communities First programme in Wales, which aimed to enhance the 'voices' of people living mainly on council estates on how to improve on their environment and public facilities. However, even though their voices were heard, they had no influence on council budgets, service delivery or prioritisation of issues. As a result, the Welsh government decided to commission research into the scheme, which prompted members of the public to recommend greater empowerment to seek out activities that improve personal health, wellbeing and personal development (Arad Research, 2017). The Welsh government has now decided to close the current programme and, from 2018, to concentrate on a scheme with a sharper focus on helping people into work and ensuring people's voices are heard when designing local services.

Woodall and colleagues (2010) concluded that: (a) any noticeable change following an individual or community empowerment programme may not be solely due to the empowering approach; and (b) a more transparent and mutually agreed definition of 'empowerment' is needed. To these caveats can be added the need for those advocating empowerment for improved health to agree on *how* to empower people. Ironically, one could ask whether health promotion professionals themselves have the power to enable individuals and communities to bring about a change to their social and environmental conditions, when only a government – local and/or national – has the authority to bring about that change by devolving some of their own power (Gottwald and Goodman-Brown, 2012).

Research evidence and evaluation

Chapter Three discussed the process and methods of evaluation, while Chapter Five considered the range of evaluation options open to health economists in identifying whether an intervention produced value for money. Here, the discussion will focus on the basic question of whether there can ever be a solution to the apparent pessimism among health promotion analysts on the topic of health promotion evaluation.

Nutbeam's (1998) concern that 'evaluation of health promotion is a difficult enterprise which is often done poorly' is a consistent regret in the literature. Numerous scholarly articles and publications (for example, WHO, 2002; O'Connor et al., 2006; Victorian Government, 2008) pay a good deal of attention to how to create the right circumstances to clearly interpret the performance and outcomes of health promotion interventions. The WHO (2002) report runs to 561 pages but suffers from the same pervading gap in the relevant literature: there is a dearth of references to case studies that shed any light on competent evaluation techniques, or why certain health promotion programmes and projects have or have not been successful.

In addition, of those particular programmes and projects reported in the professional literature, very few relate to the UK. Of a random selection of 200 articles in the journal *Health Promotion International*, only five case studies and five systematic reviews were UK-related. A similar proportion was published in the *International Journal of Health Promotion and Education*. One reason for this is that the commissioning agency (such as a government department) does not often publish the evaluation findings in a wider context than an internal report (Palfrey et al., (2012). Another possible reason for the lack of research-based evidence on the success of health promotion is that health promotion is a complex endeavour, the outcomes of which might not emerge until after a lengthy stretch of time. Both of these 'excuses' are open to challenge. First, every health promotion activity must have clear and articulated objectives; if it does not, then it is ill-conceived and poorly designed. Second, many health promotion interventions unavoidably take time to produce either positive or negative results that can validly be interpreted as the success or failure of the project. To post this as a problem is deceptive. The Caerphilly Cohort Study (described in Chapter Three) was evaluated during and at the end of a 30-year period and recorded a number of verifiable, validated statistics.

Nutbeam (1998) expressed typical frustration some years ago: 'It is hard to identify a simple cause chain which links a health promotion to changes in health status. ... The link between health promotion action and eventual health outcomes is usually complex and difficult to trace' (p 35). As an example, Nutbeam cites attempts to quit, or not start, smoking: 'Even here, where the link between a behaviour and health outcome is established, the relationship between different forms of health promotion intervention – education, behavioural counselling, changing social attitudes, environmental restrictions and price increases – and subsequent decision by an individual to quit or not to start, are very complex' (p 35).

If those mounting a health promotion activity want to find out why some people stopped smoking, reduced their smoking habit or went on to vaping, a possibly facetious suggestion is: *Ask them.* Reports of health promotion evaluations where the intended beneficiaries are asked for feedback are few and far between. There is hardly any point in attempting to help people maintain, manage or improve their health if the programme does not have an acceptable method of discovering how effective it has been, and the reasons why it has succeeded or failed, built into it. Part of this method of assessment should be to check how the intervention is proceeding towards its stated objective(s). This involves evaluating the stage of evaluation known as **process**.

Hubley and Copeman (2013) list six steps to be followed in designing the evaluation:

1 Set SMART (specific, measurable, achievable, realistic and time-scaled) objectives at the beginning of the programme.
2 Carry out a baseline study to be able to demonstrate any changes as a result of the programme's activities.
3 Address process, outcome and impact, and look for achievements as well as programme failures in the design of the evaluation.

4 If possible, identify controls (identical or similar situations) to be able to show change as a result of the programme activities.
5 Involve all partners in the evaluation.
6 Plan to record any programme benefits that might otherwise be missed by the evaluation; for example, 'spin-offs' such as an increase in community cohesion.

One way of enhancing the chances of being able to identify whether the programme has been a success is to involve all partners not only in the evaluation but also at the outset, when designing the health promotion programme. The wealth of literature on empowering people seems reluctant to state exactly *how* this is to be achieved, other than helping them to develop 'skills' to take more control of their lives. Ensuring that people contribute at the earliest stage in a health promotion programme tells them their views are valued and offers a clearer opportunity for them to improve their self-esteem. This approach is labelled a **bottom-up** style of evaluation; it is clearly distinguished from a **top-down** approach, in which the health promoter 'expert' judges whether the programme or project has been a success (Laverack, 2014):

> A bottom-up style of evaluation places the focus on involving all the partners through participatory methods and moves practice away from conventional 'expert'-driven approaches. This means a fundamental shift between the practitioners and the beneficiaries of the programme, one where control over decisions about the evaluation are more equitably distributed. The evaluation helps to empower the beneficiaries by actively involving them in the process of evaluation and skills development to subsequently provide the means to improve the programme further. (Laverack, 2007, quoted in Laverack, 2014, p 113)

It must be acknowledged that carrying out a randomised controlled trial within the context of a health promotion initiative would be extremely difficult, for reasons discussed in Chapter Three. To test whether the intervention has proved successful, other evaluation methods would therefore have to rely primarily on other data collection techniques. Palfrey et al. (2012) set down a range of such techniques, each of which has its own strengths and potential limitations:

- in-depth interviews – individual or in groups
- observation – participant and nonparticipant
- survey of documents
- questionnaires
- natural experiments

A combination of two or more data collection methods, known as **triangulation**, would be most likely to generate data that would rate as 'highly probable' as an indication of the intervention's effectiveness. This criterion does not necessarily apply only to the project's outcomes. An assessment of its process – for example, in persuading people to take part in the programme or project; in providing ongoing feedback on the project's implementation and whether changes to the intended objective(s) or period of the intervention were required – would provide extremely useful information on the reasons for the degree of the programme's success. Given the range of options health promotion practitioners and managers have for delivering research-based evidence, it is puzzling why regrets about the 'complexity' of health promotion and lack of research evidence have persisted over such a length of time.

The future for health promotion

The case against

Three of the global conferences referenced in the previous chapter claimed that health promotion was effective and cost-effective, and reduced inequities and poverty. These claims were not backed up by clear evidence. This exemplifies one of the central criticisms of health promotion: over the decades in which it has been a key public health strategy, there is little evidence that it has made significant changes in either people's health behaviours or their capacity or willingness to adopt a healthier lifestyle. At the heart of any efforts to help individuals and communities avoid suffering illnesses is the concept of empowerment, discussed throughout this book. The prevailing rationale for this approach is to help people take control over their lives so they can choose options that are health-giving rather than those that are health risky (Matthews, 1999). Health promotion, it is argued, can enable people to develop skills that will guide them towards making the 'right' choices. However, exactly what these 'skills' are remain obscure. This leads to another criticism: that this strategy is indicative of the nanny state syndrome that strives to impose middle-class values on the rest of the population. It is evident that, over the centuries, governments in the UK have regarded healthy citizenship as contributing to national economic stability and development through maintaining a healthy workforce. Yet, in terms of health promotion leading to a reduction in NHS expenditure, there is no hard evidence that health promotion does indeed achieve a reduction. If people are not taking steps to improve their health or avoid becoming unhealthy, they are seen as guilty of 'letting the country down' – not just themselves.

Those who espouse the 'social determinants of health' explanation of how some sections of the population have higher rates of morbidity and mortality than others would regard the approach of trying to help some people make 'healthier choices' as misguided and doomed to failure. There would appear to be conclusive evidence that people experiencing low income, poor housing and long-term unemployment are more likely to be susceptible to illness – both physical and mental – than those who do not suffer from these disadvantages. To label these as 'social determinants' could be said to be inaccurate. Low income, poor housing and long-term unemployment are determined by economic and political decisions, not by whatever 'social' is meant to convey. To galvanise people in groups – or 'communities', to use the accepted nomenclature – to challenge these determinants is outside the scope of health promotion practitioners.

The case in favour

There is some evidence that schools-based health promotion activities have proved successful, particularly in the field of mental health (Pybis et al., 2012; Rupani et al., 2012; Cooper, 2013;). Programmes in schools are implementing the basic premise of health promotion, which is to intervene at an early stage in the life cycle to prevent health problems happening later on. However, as noted in Chapter Six, a number of charitable organisations have the primary objective of carrying out mental health promotion in schools.

Recently, a health promotion initiative launched by GPs in England promises to show successful health outcomes. As reported in *The Times* (Bee, 2017), about 100,000 more overweight people a year will be offered NHS exercise and cookery classes as a result of GP referrals. The scheme is designed to ward off type 2 diabetes and save money for the NHS in the long term. GPs offer blood tests and 13-class courses on healthy eating and keeping fit to those they consider most at risk. The uptake to date has been very encouraging. Similar schemes around the world have been shown to cut new diabetes cases by about a quarter. Global conferences have expressed worldwide agreement that an intersectoral approach would be the most effective way of designing and implementing health promotion policies and programmes. This would enable a more comprehensive strategy, which would seek to reduce health inequalities through action at all government levels.

The verdict

Under the aegis of the NHS public health trusts across the UK, health promotion interventions have produced very little research-based evidence that they have made or are making progress in improving people's health. The main reason given for this is the need to monitor and evaluate programmes and projects over a lengthy period of time. This is especially the case where even a noticeable positive outcome may not be sustainable as an eventual impact. To make a convincing argument for further funding over the next 20 years, health promotion agencies in the statutory sector would need to present a portfolio of projects with a truly participatory, bottom-up design and method of evaluation. The NHS in England, Scotland, Wales and Northern Ireland need to engage in constructive conversations with both LAs and health promotion charities as to the part they can play in a 20-year health promotion programme. NHS resources are scarce enough; they should not be allocated to services that, however worthy in intent, cannot prove their effectiveness.

References

Aceijas, C (2011) *Assessing evidence to improve public health and well-being*, Exeter: Learning Matters.

Acheson Report (1998) *Independent inquiry into inequalities in health*, London: The Stationery Office.

Adams, J (2006) The failure of seat-belt legislation, in M Verweij, and M Thompson, (eds) *Clumsy solutions for a complex world*, London: Palgrave Macmillan, 132-154.

Aldermann, A (2013) *Evidence for health: From patient choice to global policy*, Cambridge: Cambridge University Press.

All Wales Mental Health Promotion Network (2010) *Promoting mental health and preventing mental illness*, www.wales.nhs.uk/news/15934.

Alzheimers Society (2017) *Alzheimers disease*, www.alzheimers.org.uk.

Andermann, A (2013) *Evidence for health: From patient choice to global policy*, Cambridge: Cambridge University Press.

Appleby, J (2016) *How does NHS spending compare with health spending internationally?* London: King's Fund.

Arad Research (2017) *Communities First: lessons learnt Welsh Government*, www.assembly.wales.

Armstrong, E (1993) Promoting mental health, in A Dines and A Cribb (eds) *Health promotion: Concepts and practice*, Oxford: Blackwell, 93–109.

Ashton, J and Seymour, H (1988) *The new public health: The Liverpool experience*, Milton Keynes: Open University Press.

Audit Scotland (2016) *The NHS in Scotland October 2016*, Edinburgh: Scottish Government.

BACP (British Association for Counselling and Psychotherapy) (2013) *School-based counselling: What is it and why we need it*, www.bcp.co.uk.

Baggott, R (2000) *Public health: Policy and politics*, Basingstoke: Palgrave Macmillan.

Baggott, R (2004) *Health and health care in Britain*, Basingstoke: Palgrave Macmillan.

Baldock, J, Manning, M, Miller, S and Vickerstaff, S (1999) *Social policy*, Oxford: Oxford University Press.

Barnardo's (2016) *It doesn't happen here*, London: Barnardo's.

Barrow, M (2012) Campaigns to persuade the nation to adopt a healthier diet are failing, *The Times*, 26 July, p 15.

Bartrip, P (1996) *Themselves writ large: The BMA 1832–1966*, London: BMJ.

Bates, S (2008) National Archives: Police opposed seat belt laws as waste of their time, *The Guardian*, 1 August, www.theguardian.com/uk/2008/aug/01/nationalarchives.police.

BBC Wales (2017) *Investigation into River Teifi pollution incident in Lampeter*, 6 June, www.bbc.co.uk/news/aav/uk-wales-40180914/river-teifi-pollution-difficult-to-investigate.

Bee, P (2017) Health classes for overweight prove a big hit, *The Times*, 17 June, p 7.

Bennett, P and Murphy, S (2001) *Psychology and health promotion*, Buckingham: Open University Press.

Bentham, J (1789) *An Introduction to the principles of morals and legislation*, London: T. Payne.

Berridge, V (2010) Historical and policy approaches to the evaluation of health promotion, in M Thorogood and Y Coombes, *Evaluating health promotion: Practice and methods*, Oxford: Oxford University Press, 11–22.

Berridge, V and Loughlin, K (2005) Smoking and the new health education in Britain 1950s–1970s, *American Journal of Public Health*, 95, 6, 956–64.

Bevan, A (1949) *Speech on the second reading of the NHS Bill*, House of Commons debate, vol. 461 cols 1448–61, 17 February.

Bevan, A (1952) *In place of fear: A free health service*, London: Heinemann.

Black Report (1980) *Inequalities in health*, London: DHSS.

Blane, D, Smith, DG and Bartley, M (1990) Social class differences in years of potential life lost: Size, trends and principal causes, *British Medical Journal*, 301, 29–32.

Booth, C (1903) *Life and labour of the people of London*, London: Macmillan and Co.

Borowitz, M and Sheldon, T (1993) Controlling health care: From economic interventions to micro-clinical regulation, *Health Economics*, 2, 201–4.

Boyce, T, Robertson, R and Dixon, A (2008) *Commissioning and behaviour change: Kicking bad habits*, London: The King's Fund.

Breslow, L (1990) A health promotion primer for the 1990s, *Home Affairs*, Summer, 98–109.

British Pathé (1947) 'Coughs and Sneezes Spread Diseases', British Pathé, Issued 11 December 1947, www.britishpathe. com/video/coughs-sneezes-spread-diseases.

Byford, S, Harrington, R, Torgerson, D, Kerfoot, M, Dyer, E, Harrington, V, Woodham, A, Gill, J, McNiven, F (1999) Cost-effectiveness analysis of a home-based social work intervention for children and adolescents who have deliberately poisoned themselves, *British Journal of Psychiatry*, 4, 56–62.

Cairns, J (1995) The costs of prevention, *British Medical Journal*, 311, 1520.

Calouste Gulbenkian Foundation (1984) *A national centre for community development: Report of a working party*, London: Grubb Foundation.

Campbell, BMS (1991) *Before the Black Death: Studies in the 'crises' of the early 14th century*, Manchester: Manchester University Press.

Carrington, D (2017) UK's new air pollution plan dismissed as 'weak' and 'woefully inadequate', *The Guardian*, 5 May, www. theguardian.com/environment/2017/may/05/government-fails-to-commit-to-diesel-scrappage-scheme-in-uk-clean-air-plan.

Carter, N, Klein, R and Day, P (1992) *How organizations measure success: The use of performance indicators in government*, London: Routledge.

Centers for Disease Control and Prevention (2014) *National prevention strategy: America's plan for better health and wellness*, Atlanta, GA: CDC.

Chadwick, E (1842) *Report on the sanitary conditions of the labouring population of Great Britain*, London: Poor Law Commission.

Chambers Dictionary (2014) London: Chambers Harrap.

Charities Evaluation Services (1998) *Involving users in evaluation*, London: CES.

Chiuve, SE McCullough, MI, Sacks, FM and Rimm, EB, (2006) Healthy lifestyle factors in the primary prevention of coronary heart disease among men, *Circulation*, 114, 160–7.

Child Poverty Action Group (2016) *Child poverty facts and figures*, London: CPAG.

Chitsabesan, P, Kroll, L, Bailey, S, Kenning, C, Sneider, S, MacDonald, W, and Theodosiou, L (2006) Mental health needs of young offenders in custody and in the community, *British Journal of Psychiatry*, 188, 6, 534–40.

Christiansen, R (2007) The story behind the hymn, *The Daily Telegraph*, 22 September, www.telegraph.co.uk/culture/music/3668062/The-story-behind-the-hymn.html.

CHRODIS (2015) *Health promotion and primary prevention in 14 European countries*, http://chrodis.eu/wp-content/uploads/2015/07/FinalFinalSummaryofWP5CountryReports.pdf.

Chu, C, Breucker, G, Harris, V, Stitzel, A, Gan, X, Gu, X and Dwyer, S (2000) Health-promoting workplaces, *Health Promotion International*, 15, 2, 155–67.

Clarke, A (1999) *Evaluation research: An introduction to principles, methods and practice*, London: Sage.

Coast, J, Donovan, K and Frankel, S (eds) (1996) *Priority setting and the healthcare debate*, Chichester: Wiley.

Coates, K and Silburn, R (1970) *Poverty: The forgotten Englishmen* London: Penguin.

Cochrane, A (1972) *Effectiveness and efficiency: Random reflections on health services*, London: Nuffield Provincial Hospital Trust.

Cohen, BI (1984) Florence Nightingale, *Scientific American*, March, 250 (3), 128–37.

Cohen, D and Hale, J (2003) The economics of health and health improvement, in Bunton, R and Macdonald, G (eds) *Health promotion: Discipline and diversity*, London: Routledge, 178–96.

Coles, E, Themessl-Huber, M, and Freeman, R (2012) Investigating community-based health and health promotion: A mixed methods review, *Health Education Research*, 27, 4, 624–44.

Cooper, M (2013) *School-based counselling in UK secondary schools: A review and critical evaluation*, Glasgow: University of Strathclyde.

Coote, A (1997) *User involvement in health care: Where next?* The Association of Charitable Foundations Fourth Annual Lecture on Philanthropy, London: King's Fund.

Cootes, RJ (1967) *The making of the welfare state*, London: Longmans, Green & Co.

Cowley, P (2009) *Where did it all go right?* [TV programme] Channel 8: BBC News.

Cragg, L, Davies, M and Macdowell, W (2013) *Health promotion theory*, Buckinghamshire: Open University Press.

Creighton, C (1965) *A history of epidemics vol. 2*, London: Frank Cass.

Davey, B and Popay, J (1993) *Dilemmas in health care*, Buckingham: Open University Press.

Davies, J, and Kelly, M (eds) (1992) *Healthy cities: Policy and practice*, London: Routledge.

Davies, JK and Macdonald, G (1998) *Quality, evidence and effectiveness in health promotion*, London: Routledge.

Declaration of Alma Ata (1978) International Conference on primary healthcare, Alma Ata, USSR 6-12 September.

Dementia UK (2017) *About dementia*, www.dementiauk.org/ understanding-dementia/about-dementia.

Department of Health (1976) *Prevention and health: Everybody's business*, London: HMSO.

Department of Health (1992) *Health of the nation*, London: DOH.

Department of Health (1995) *Variations in health: What can the Department of Health and the NHS do?* London: DOH.

Department of Health (1999) *Our healthier nation*, London: DOH.

Department of Health (2001) *Changing the outlook: A strategy for developing and modernising mental health services in prison*, London: DOH.

Department of Health (2006) *Our health, our care, our say*, cmnd 6737, London: DOH.

Department of Health (2008) *Taking the lead: Engaging people and communities* London: DoH.

Department of Health Northern Ireland (2014) *Connected health economy*, Belfast: NI Direct.

Department of Health Northern Ireland (2016) *A fitter future for all: Outcome framework 2015–2019*, Belfast: NI Direct.

DHSS (1976) *Prevention and Health: Everybody's Business*, London: HMSO.

Dines, A and Cribb, A (eds) (1993) *Health promotion: Concepts and practice*, Oxford: Blackwell.

Dixey, R, Cross, R, Foster, S, Lowcock, D, Smith, J, Warwick-Booth, L, White, J and Woodall, J (2012) *Health promotion: Global principles and practice*, Oxford: CABI.

Doll, R and Hill, AB (1950) Smoking and carcinoma of the lung, *BMJ*, 2, 4682, 739–48.

Drever, F and Bunting, J (1997) Patterns and trends in male mortality, in Drever, F and Whitehead, M (eds) *Health inequalities: Decennial supplement*, London: Stationery Office, 95–107.

Dreverm, M and Whitehead, M (eds) (1997) *Health inequalities*, London: Stationery Office.

Drummond, MF, Sculpher, MJ and Torrance, GW (2005) *Methods for the evaluation of healthcare programmes*, Oxford: Oxford University Press.

Drummond, M, Weatherly, H, Claxton, K, Cookson, R, Ferguson, B, Godfrey, C, Rice, N, Sculpher, M and Snowden, A (2007) *Assessing the challenges of applying standard methods of economic evaluation to public health interventions*, York: Public Health Research Consortium.

Edwards, N (2014) *Community services: How they can transfer care*, London: King's Fund.

Elwood, P, Galante, J, Pickering J, Palmer, S, Bayer, A, Ben-Shiomo, Y, Longley, M and Gallacher, J (2013) Healthy lifestyles reduce the incidence of chronic disease and dementia: Evidence from the Caerphilly Cohort Study, *Public Library of Science*, 8, 12, 9 December.

Ewles, L and Simnett, J (2003) *Health promotion: Practical approaches*, London: Elsevier Health Services.

Faculty of Public Health (2010) *Better mental health for all*, www.fph.org.uk/a_good_start_in_life.

Farr, W (1839) Letter to the Registrar General, *First annual report of the Registrar General*, London: HMSO.

Farr, W (1864) Letter to the Registrar General, *Supplement to the 25th annual report of the Registrar General for the years 1851–1860*, London: HMSO.

Fetterman, DM (1994) Empowerment evaluation, *Evaluation Practice*, 15, 1, 1–15.

Fetterman, DM, Kattarian, AJ and Wandersman, A (eds) (1995) *Empowerment evaluation: Knowledge tools for self-assessment and accountability*, London: Sage.

Fitzpatrick, T (2001) *Welfare theory: An introduction*, Basingstoke: Palgrave.

Ford, ES, Zhao, G, Tsai, J and Li, C (2011) Low-risk lifestyle behaviours and all-cause mortality, *American Journal of Public Health*, 17 October vol 101, 10, 1922–9.

Foundation for People with Learning Disabilities (2017) *Learning disability statistics and mental health problems*, www.mentalhealth.org.uk/learning-disabilities/help-information/learning-disability-statistics-/187699.

Fowler, PBS (1997) Evidence-based everything, *Journal of Evaluation in Clinical Practice*, 3, 3, 239–43.

Fox, KR (1999) The influence of physical activity on mental well-being, *Public Health Nutrition*, 2, 3a, 411–18.

Franceschini, MC and Rice, M (2011) *Advancing health promotion in the Americas*, Pan American Health Organization.

Frankish, CJ, Hwang, SW and Quantz, D (2005) Homelessness and health in Canada, *Canadian Journal of Public Health*, March/April, 96, 523–9.

Fried, A and Elman, R (eds) (1971) *Charles Booth's London*, London: Penguin.

Friedli, L and Parsonage, M (2009) *Promoting mental health and preventing mental illness: The economic case for investment in Wales*, Cardiff: All Wales Health Promotion Network.

Gazely, I (2003) *Poverty in Britain 1900–1945*, London: Palgrave Macmillan.

Gibbon, M (2000) The health analysis and action cycle: An empowering approach to women's health, *Sociological Research Online*, 4, 4, www.socresonline.org.uk/4/4/gibbon.html.

Gimpel, J (2015) A third of children in England are overweight/obese, *Archives of disease in childhood*, London: King's College.

Glouberman, S and Millar, J (2003) Evolution of the determinants of health, health policy and health information systems in Canada, *American Journal of Public Health*, 93, 3, 388–92.

Gottwald, M and Goodman-Brown, J (2012) *A guide to practical health promotion*, Maidenhead: Open University Press.

Green, J and Thorogood, N (1998) *Analysing health policy: A sociological approach*, London: Longman.

Green, J and Tones, K (2012) *Health promotion planning and strategies*, London: Sage.

Green, L (1979) National policy on the promotion of health, *International Journal of Health Education*, 22, 161–8.

Greenhalgh, T (1997) *How to read a paper: The basis of evidence-based medicine*, London: British Medical Journal Publishing.

Gregson, RJ and Court, LA (2010) *Building health communities: A community empowerment approach*, London: Community Development Foundation.

Guba, EG and Lincoln, YS (1989) *Fourth generation evaluation*, Newbury Park, CA: Sage.

Hubley, J and Copeman, J (2008) *Practical health promotion*, Cambridge: Polity Press.

Haddad, L, Cameron, L and Bennett, I (2015) The double burden of malnutrition in S E Asia and the Pacific: Priorities, policies and politics, *Health Policy Planning*, 30, 9, 1193–206.

Hale, J (2000) What contribution can health economics make to health promotion? *Health Promotion International*, 15, 4, 341–8.

Hale, J, Phillips, CJ and Jewell, T (2012) Making the economic case for prevention: A view from Wales, *Public Health*, 12, 460.

Halliday, S (2000) William Farr: Campaigning statistician, *Journal of Medical Biography*, 8, 4, 220–7.

Hamilton-Shield, MP (2014) Childhood obesity: What harm, any solutions, in Haslam, D, Sharma, AM and le Roux, CW (eds), *Controversies in obesity*, London: Springer, 214–16.

Hann, A (ed) (2000) *Analysing health policy*, Aldershot: Ashgate.

Harris, JB, LaRocque, RC, Qadri, F, Ryan, ET and Calderwood, SB (2012) Cholera, *The Lancet*, 379, 9835, 2466–76.

Harvey, I (1996) Philosophical perspectives in priority setting, in Coast, J, Donovan, K and Frankel, S (eds) *Priority setting and the healthcare debate*, Chichester: Wiley, 83–110.

Haslam, D, Sharma, AM and le Roux, CW (2014) *Controversies in obesity*, London: Springer.

Health and Social Care Information Centre (2016) *Statistics on obesity, physical activity and diet: England*, London: HSCIC.

Health and Social Care Public Health Agency Northern Ireland (2013) *Major campaign to tackle obesity*, Belfast: HSCPHA.

Health Canada (2005) *Health promotion*, www.med.uottawa.ca/ sim/data/health_promotion_e.htm.

Health Foundation, The (2017) *Healthy lives for people in the UK*, London: Health Foundation.

Hodgkinson, R (1967) *The origins of the NHS: The medical services of the new Poor Law*, London: Wellcome Foundation.

Hodgkiss, A (2001) Mental health problems alongside physical illness, in Ramsay, R, Gerada, C, Mars, S and Szmukler, G, *Mental illness: A handbook for carers*, London: Jessica Kingsley, 89–96.

Hollis, P (1974) *Pressure from without in early Victorian England*, London: Edward Arnold.

HomelessLink (2017) *Homelessness in numbers*, www.homeless. org.uk/facts/homelessness-in-numbers.

Honigsbaum, F (1970) *The struggle for the Ministry of Health*, London: Social Administration Research Trust.

How prejudiced is the NHS? (2017) [TV programme] BBC 2: BBC.

Howard, J (1777) *The state of prisons in England and Wales*, Warrington: Cadell and Conant.

Hubley, J and Copeman, J (2013) *Practical health promotion*, Cambridge: Polity Press.

Hudson, M (2016) *The management of mental health at work*, London: ACAS.

Hughes, L (2016) More spent on treating obesity-related conditions than on the police or fire service, says NHS chief, *The Telegraph*, 7 June, www.telegraph.co.uk/news/2016/06/07/ more-spent-on-treating-obesity-related-conditions-than-on-the-po/.

IAS (Institute of Alcohol Studies) (2016) *The economic impacts of alcohol*, www.ias.org.uk.

Illich, I (1974) *Medical nemesis: The expropriation of health*, London: Calder and Boyars.

IMF (International Monetary Fund) (2017) *Civil Society and the IMF*, Washington: IMF.

Institute for Health Metrics and Evaluation (2017) *Conflicts subverting improvements to health conditions in the Eastern Mediterranean region*, Seattle, WA: University of Washington.

Johnston, I (2014) Children taken into care for being too fat, *The Independent*, 28 February, www.independent.co.uk/life-style/health-and-families/health-news/children-taken-into-care-for-being-too-fat-9158809.html.

Joint Commissioning Panel for Mental Health (2013) *Guidance for commissioning for mental health services for people with learning disabilities*, www.jcpmh.info.

Joseph Rowntree Foundation (2008) *The cost of child poverty for individuals and society*, Save the Children website, www.jrf.org.uk/sites/default/files/jrf/migrated/files/2301-child-poverty-costs.pdf.

Kelly, A and Symonds, A (2003) *The social construction of community nursing*, London: Palgrave Macmillan.

Kelly, J (2011) How high-visibility took over Britain, *BBC News*, 30 August, www.bbc.co.uk/news/magazine-14720101.

Khan, L and Wilson, J (2010) You just get on and do it: Healthcare provision, *Youth Offending Team*, www.centreformentalhealth.org.uk.

Khaw, KT, Wareham, N, Bingham, S and Luben, R (2008) Combined impact of health behaviours and mortality in men and women, *Public Library of Science Medicine*, 5, 3, e70.

Killoran, A and Kelly, MP (eds) (2010) *Evidence-based public health*, Oxford: Oxford University Press.

Kilner, JF (1990) *Who lives? Who Dies? Ethical criteria in patient selection*, New Haven, CT: Yale University Press.

King's Fund (2017a) *Health inequalities*, 23 March, www.kingsfund.org.uk/projects/nhs-in-a-nutshell/health-inequalities.

King's Fund (2017b) *Transforming our healthcare system*, www.kingsfund.org.uk.

Koelen, MA and Lindstrom, B (2005) Making healthy choices easy choices: The role of empowerment, *European Journal of Clinical Nutrition*, 5a, suppl. 1, S10–S6.

Lalonde Report (1974) *A new perspective on the health of Canadians: A working document*, Ottawa: Government of Canada.

Lansley, S and Mack, J (2015) *Breadline Britain: The rise of mass poverty*, London: Oneworld.

Laverack, G (2007) *Health promotion practice: Building empowered communities*, Maidenhead: Open University Press.

Laverack, G (2009) *Health promotion practice: Power and empowerment*, London: Sage.

Laverack, G (2014) *The pocket guide to health promotion*, Maidenhead: Open University Press.

Laverack, G and Wallerstein, N (2001) Measuring community empowerment: A fresh look at organizational domains, *Health Promotion International*, 16, 179–85.

Le Fanu, J (ed) (1994) *Preventionitis: Exaggerated claims of health promotion*, British Medical Journal.

LeGrand, J (1987) Equity, health and healthcare, *Social Justice Research*, 1, 237–74.

Lewis, J (1992) Providers, Consumers: the State and the delivery of health-care services in Twentieth-Century Britain, in Wear, A (ed) *Medicine in society: historical essays*, Cambridge: Cambridge University Press, 317–45.

Lind, J (1753) *A treatise on the scurvy*, London: A. Millar.

Little, W, Fowler, HW, Coulson, J, revised and edited by Onion, CT (1933) *Shorter Oxford English Dictionary*, Oxford: Clarendon Press.

Loades, ME and Mastroyannopoulu, K (2010) Teachers' recognition of children's mental health problems, *Child and Adolescent Mental Health*, 15, 3, 150–6.

Logan, WPD (1950) Mortality in England and Wales from 1848–1947, *Population Studies*, 4, 132–78.

Longmate, N (1966) *King Cholera: The biography of a disease*, London: Hamish Hamilton.

Loy, K (2017) Parental opposition to having child vaccinated, *The Times*, 9 March, p 13.

Lumley, WG (1859) *The new sanitary law*, London: Shaw and Sons.

Macnicol, J (1998) *The politics of retirement in Britain 1908–1948*, Cambridge: Cambridge University Press.

Main, G and Bradshaw, J (2016) Child poverty in the UK: Measures, prevalence and intra-household sharing, *Critical Social Policy*, 36, 1, 38–61.

Malthus, T (1798) *An essay on the principles of population*, London: J. Johnson.

Mark, MM and Shotland, RI (1985) Stakeholder-based evaluation and value judgements, *Evaluation Review*, 9, 5, 605–26.

Marmot, M (2010) *Fair society, healthy lives: Strategic review of health inequalities in England post-2010*, London: Dept For International Development.

Marsh, K, Edwards, RT, Williams, N, Raisanen, L, Moore, G, Linck, P, Hounsome, N, Ud Din, N and Moore, L (2012a) An evaluation of the effectiveness and cost-effectiveness of the National Referral Scheme in Wales, UK: A randomised controlled trial of a public health policy initiative, *Journal of Epidemiology and Community Health*, 66, 8, 745–53.

Marsh, K, Phillips, CJ, Fordham, R, Bertranou, E and Hale, J (2012b) Estimating cost-effectiveness in public health: A summary of modelling and valuation methods, *Health Economic Review*, 2, 1, 17, www.ncbi.nlm.nih.gov/pubmed/22943762.

Mason, R (2017) UK Government agrees to publish air pollution strategy in the next week, *The Guardian*, 2 May, www.theguardian.com/environment/2017/may/02/uk-government-publish-air-pollution-strategy.

Masters, R, Anwar, E, Collins, B, Cookson, R and Capewell, S (2017) Return on investment of public health interventions: A systematic review, *Journal of Epidemiology and Public Health*, 0, 1–8.

Matthews, UN (1999) *Epidemiology and public health medicine*, London: Churchill Livingstone.

Maybin, J and Klein, R (2012) *Thinking about rationing*, London: King's Fund.

McCullough, M, Patel, AV, Kushi, LH, Patel, R and Willett, WC (2011) Following cancer prevention guidelines reduces risk of cancer, cardio-vascular disease and all-cause mortality, *Cancer Epidemiology*, 20, 1089–97.

McDonald, L (ed) (2004) *Florence Nightingale on Public Health care*, Waterloo, Canada: Wilfred Laurier University Press.

McKeown, T (1972) An interpretation of the modern rise in population in Europe, *Population Studies*, 26, 345–82.

McKeown, T (1976) *The role of medicine: Dream, mirage or nemesis?* Oxford: Blackwell.

McKeown, T (1979) *The role of medicine: dream, mirage or nemesis?* Oxford: Blackwell.

McQueen, DV and Jones, C (eds) (2007) *Global perspectives on health promotion*, New York, NY: Springer.

Meltzer, H, Gadward, R, Goodman, R and Ford, T (2000) *The mental health of children and adolescents in Great Britain*, London: ONS.

Mental Health Act 1983, c.20, London: HMSO.

Mental Health Foundation (2016a) *Mental health in Northern Ireland: Fundamental facts*, www.mentalhealth.org.uk.

Mental Health Foundation (2016b) *Mental Health in Wales: Fundamental facts* www.mentalhealth.org.uk.

Mental Health Foundation (2017) www.mentalhealth.org.uk.

Mental Health Taskforce to the NHS in England (2016) *The five year forward View for mental health*, London: England.

Merrison Report (1979) *Report of the Royal Commission on the NHS*, London: HMSO.

Merton, RK (1957) *Social theory and social structure*, Glencoe, IL: Free Press.

Mill, JS (1860) *On liberty*, London: Longman, Roberts and Green.

Mind (2016) *Our communities; our mental health: Commissioning for better mental health*, London: Mind.

Ministry of Health (1981) *Public health propaganda: Smoking and lung cancer's publicity policy (1957–60)*, National Archives, MH 55/2203.

Mold, A and Berridge, V (2013) *The history of health promotion*, London: McGraw-Hill.

Moody, O. (2015) Report of the National children's bureau, *The Times*, 7 September, p 7.

Murphy, SM, Edwards, RT, Williams, N, Raisanen, L, Moore, G and Iunck, P (2012) An evaluation of the effectiveness and cost-effectiveness of the National Exercise Referral Scheme in Wales, UK: A randomised controlled trial of a public health policy initiative, *Journal of Epidemiology Community Health*, 46, 8, 745–53.

Musson, AE (1959) The Great Depression in Britain 1973–1896: A reappraisal, *International Journal of Economic History*, 19, 2, 199–228.

Naidoo, B (2010) Evaluating the use of public health risk factors simulation, in Thorogood, M and Coombes, Y (eds) *Evaluating health promotion practice and methods*, Oxford: Oxford University Press, 98–109.

Naidoo, J and Wills, J (2016) *Foundations for health promotion*, Kidlington: Elsevier.

National Audit Office (2001) *Tackling obesity in England*, London: NAO.

National Children's Bureau (2015) *Poor beginnings: Health inequalities among young children across England*, London: NCB.

National Diet and nutrition Survey (2016) *The diet, nutrition and nutritional status of the general population of the UK*, Public Health England, www.gov.uk/government/collections/national-diet-and-nutrition-survey.

National Social Marketing Centre (2016) *Alcohol*, www.thensmc/resources/vfm/alcohol.

Nettleton, S (1992) *Power, pain and dentistry*, Buckingham: Open University Press.

NICE (National Institute for Health and Care Excellence) (2011) *Supporting investment in public health: Review of methods for assessing the cost-effectiveness, cost impact and returns on investment*, London: NICE.

NICE (2016) *Mental health problems in people with learning disabilities: Prevention, assessment and management*, www.nice.org.uk?guidance/ng54.

Noblet, A and LaMOntagne, AD (2006) The role of workplace health promotion in addressing job stress, *Health Promotion International*, 21, 4, 346–53.

Northern Ireland Executive (2016) *Budget 2016–17*, Belfast: NIE.

Norton, R (2016) There is no sector more important than health, *Healthcare Asia magazine*, April, http://healthcareasiamagazine.com/healthcare/feature/there-no-sector-more-important-health-pwc.

Nutbeam, D (1998) Evaluating health promotion: Progress, problems and solutions, *Health Promotion International*, 13, 1, 27-44.

Nutbeam, D (2000) Health literacy as a public health goal: A challenge for contemporary health education and communication strategy into the 21st century, *Health Promotion International*, 15, 3, 259–67.

O'Brien, L and O'Leary, J (2015) Does smoking cost as much as it makes for the Treasury? *FullFact*, www.fullfact.org/health/spending-english-nhs.

O'Connor-Fleming, MA, Parker, E, Higgins, J and Gould, T (2006) A framework for evaluating health promotion programs, *Health Promotion Journal of Australia*, 17, 1, 61–6.

O'Keefe, E, Ottewill, R and Wall, A (1992) *Community Health: issues in management*, Sunderland: Business Education Publishers Limited.

O'Leary, J (2017) NHS funding, *FullFact*, 12 January, www.fullfact.org/health/spending-english-nhs.

ONS (Office of National Statistics) (2004) *Public service productivity: Health paper 1*, London: ONS.

ONS (2016) *How does UK healthcare spending compare internationally?* London: ONS.

ONS (2017) *Statistics on obesity, physical activity and diet*, briefing paper no. 3336, 20 January, London: House of Commons Library.

Painter, J and Pande, P (2013) *Reframing citizen relationships with the public sector in a time of austerity: Community empowerment in England and Scotland*, Swindon: Arts and Humanities Research Council.

Palfrey, C (2000) *Key concepts in health care policy and planning*, Basingstoke: Macmillan.

Palfrey, C, Phillips, C, Thomas, P and Edwards, D (1992) *Policy evaluation in the public sector*, Aldershot: Avebury.

Palfrey, C, Thomas, P and Phillips, CJ (2012) *Evaluation for the real world*, Bristol: Policy Press.

Parsonage, M, Khoniou, H, Rutherford, M, Sidhu, M and Smith, C (2009) *Diversion: A better way for criminal justice and mental health*, London: Sainsbury Centre for Mental Health.

Pawson, R and Tilley, N (1997) *Realistic evaluation*, London: Sage.

Pereira, J (1993) What does equity in health mean? *Journal of Social Policy*, 22, 1, 19–48.

Petrou, S, Cooper, P, Murray, L and Davidson LL (2006) Cost-effectiveness of a preventive counselling and support package for post natal depression, *International Journal of Health Technology Assessment in Health Care*, 22, 4, 443–53.

Phillimore, P, Beattie, A and Townsend, P (1994) Widening inequality in health in northern England 1981–1991, *British Medical Journal*, 308, 1125–8.

Phillips, CJ (1997) *Economic evaluation in health promotion*, Aldershot: Avebury.

Phillips, CJ (2005) *Health economics: An introduction for health professionals*, Oxford: Blackwell.

Potvin, L and Jones, CM (2011) Twenty-five years after the Ottawa Charter: The critical role of health promotion for public health, *Canadian Journal of Public Health*, 102, 4, 244–8.

Potvin, L and McQueen, D (eds) (2008) *Health promotion practices in the Americas*, New York: Springer.

Power, R, French, R, Connelly, J, George, S, Hawes, D, Hinton, T, Klee, H, Robinson, D, Senior, J, Timms, P and Warner D (1999) Health, health promotion and homelessness, *British Medical Journal*, 318, 590–2.

Prisons and Probation Ombudsman (2016) *Mental health in prisons*, London: OGL.

Probst, C, Roerecke, M, Behrendt, R and Rehm, J (2014) Socio-economic differences in alcohol attributable mortality compared with all-cause mortality: A systematic review and meta-analysis, *International Journal of Epidemiology*, 43, 4, 1314–27.

Public Health England (2016) *Annual report and accounts 2015/16*, London: PHE.

Public Health Wales (2016a) *Making a difference: Investing in sustainable health and well-being for the people of Wales*, Cardiff: Public Health Wales NHS Trust.

Public Health Wales (2016b) *Obesity*, Cardiff: Welsh Government.

Public Health Wales (2017) *Child measurement programme for Wales*, Cardiff: Public Health Wales.

Pybis, J, Hill, A, Cooper, M, Smith, K, Maybanks, M, Cromarty, K, Pattison, S and Couchman, K (2012) A comparative analysis of the attitudes of key stakeholder groups to the Welsh Government's school-based counselling strategy, *British Journal of Guidance and Counselling*, 40, 5, 485–98.

Pyper, D and Dar, A (2015) *Zero-hours contracts*, London: House of Commons Library.

Ramsay, R, Gerada, C, Mars, S and Szmukler, G (2001) *Mental illness: A handbook for carers*, London: Jessica Kingsley.

Raphael, D (2002) *Poverty, income, inequality and health in Canada*, Toronto: CSJ Foundation for Research and Education.

Raphael, D (2008) Social determinants of health: An overview of concepts and issues, in Bryant, T, Raphael, D and Rioux, M *Staying alive: Critical perspectives on health, illness and health care*, Toronto: Canadian Scholars Press.

Rappaport, J (1987) Terms of empowerment: Exemplars of prevention, *American Journal of Community Psychology*, 15, 2, 121–48.

RCP Report (1962) *Smoking and health,* London: Pitman Medical Publishing.

Reed, J (2003) Mental health care in prisons, *British Journal of Psychiatry*, 182, 4, 287–8.

Reed Report (1992) *Review of Health and Social Services for mentally disordered offenders: final summary report*, Department of Health and Home Office Cmnd 2088, London: HM Stationery Office.

Reeves, MJ and Rafferty, AP (2005) Healthy lifestyle characteristics among adults in the United States, 2000, *Archives of International Medicine*, 165, 8, 854–7.

Regional Director (2016) *The work of the WHO in the African region*, Brazzaville, Congo: WHO.

Rey, O (2010) The use of external assessments on the impact on education, *CIDREE Yearbook*, http://cidree.org/publications/yearbook 2010/.

Richardson, A (2009) *Investing in public health*, New Zealand: Canterbury District Health Board.

Rissel, C (1994) Empowerment: The holy grail of health promotion? *Journal of Health Promotion*, 9, 1, 39–47.

ROSPA (2017) *Road Safety Factsheet: seat belts: advice and information*, Birmingham: The Royal Society for the Prevention of Accidents, www.rospa.com/rospaweb/docs/advice-services/road-safety/vehicles/seatbelt-advice.pdf.

Rowntree, BS (1901) *Poverty: A study in town life*, London: Macmillan and Co.

Runciman, WG (1966) *Relative deprivation and social justice*, London: Routledge and Kegan Paul.

Rupani, P, Cooper, M and McArthur, K (2012) A study of client goals and goal achievement within school-based counselling, *British Psychology Society Annual Conference*, Leicester.

Sabia, S, Nabi, H, Kivimaki, M. Shipley, MJ, Marmot, MG and Singh-Manoux, A (2009) Health behaviours from early to midlife as predictors of cognitive function: The Whitehall Study, *American Journal of Epidemiology*, 170, 428–37.

Sackett, DL, Rosenberg, WMC, Gray, JAM, Haynes, RB and Richardson, WS (1996) Evidence-based medicine: What it is and what it isn't, *British Medical Journal*, 312, 71.

Sainsbury Centre for Mental Health (2007) *Mental health at work: Developing the business case*, London: SCMH.

Sari, N, Castro, S and Newman, FL (2008) Should we invest in suicide prevention programs? *Journal of Socio-Economics*, 37, 262–75.

Save the Children (2012) *Child poverty in snapshots: The local picture in Wales*, Cardiff: Save the Children, https://resourcecentre.savethechildren.net/sites/default/files/documents/7137.pdf.

Scarlett, M and Denvir, J (2016) *Health survey (NI): First results*, Belfast: Department of Health.

Scott, D (2001) Qualitative approaches to the evaluation of health promotion activities, in Scott, D and Weston, R (eds) *Evaluating health promotion*, Cheltenham: Nelson Thrones, 31–48.

Scottish Government (2010a) *Equally well review*, Edinburgh: Scottish Government.

Scottish Government (2010b) *Preventing overweight and obesity in Scotland: A route map towards healthy weight*, Edinburgh: Scottish Government.

Scottish Government (2012) *Mental health strategy for Scotland 2012–2015*, Edinburgh: Scottish Government.

Scottish Government (2016a) *Obesity indicators: Monitoring progress for the prevention of obesity route*, Edinburgh: Scottish Government.

Scottish Government (2016b) *Scottish health survey*, Edinburgh: Scottish Government.

Scottish Government (2017) *Bridging the gap: Poverty and health inequalities*, Edinburgh: Scottish Government.

Scottish Public Health Observatory (2010) *Healthy weight route map: A long-term obesity strategy*, Edinburgh: ScotPHO.

Scull, A (2016) *Madness in civilization*, London: Thames and Hudson.

Searle GR (2004) *A new England*, Oxford: Oxford University Press.

Sen, A (1985) *Commodities and capabilities*, Amsterdam: North Holland.

Singleton, N, Meltzer, H and Gatward, R (1998) *Psychiatric morbidity among prisoners in England and Wales*, London: HM Stationery Office.

Small, GW, Siddarth, P, Ercoli, IM, Chen, ST and Merrill, DA (2013) Healthy behaviour and memory self-reports in young, middle-aged and older adult,' *International Psychogeriatrics*, 25, 981–9.

Small, H (1998) *Florence Nightingale: Avenging angel*, London: Constable.

Smith, K and Foster, J (2014) *Alcohol, health inequalities and the harm paradox*, London: Institute of Alcohol Studies.

Snow, T (2007) In the balance: The shift from hospitals into the community, *Nursing Standard*, 21, 34, 12–13.

Social Exclusion Unit (2002) *Report: Reducing re-offending by ex-prisoners*, London: Social Exclusion Unit.

Speers, M (1996) Encouraging trends in health promotion in the United States, *Health Promotion International*, 11, 2, 69–71.

Sperling, RA, Alsen, PS, Beckett, LA, Bennett, DA and Craft, S (2011) Towards defining the preclinical stages of Alzheimers disease, *Alzheimers Dementia*, 7, 280–91.

Spoth, R (1989) Applying conjoint analysis of consumer preferences to the development of utility-responsive health promotion programs, *Health Education Research*, 4, 439–49.

Spoth, R and Redmond, C (1993) Identifying program preferences through conjoint analysis: illustrative results from a parent sample, *American Journal of Health Promotion*, 8, 124–33.

Srivastava, D (2008) *Is prevention better than cure?* Policy brief. London: London School of Economics, http://eprints.lse. ac.uk/26162/.

Stampfer, MJ, Hu, FB, Manson, JE, Rimm, EB and Willett, WC (2000) Primary prevention of heart disease in women through diet and lifestyle, *New England Journal of Medicine*, 343, 16–22.

Stewart-Brown, S and McMillan, AS (2010 *Home and community based parenting support programmes and interventions*, Coventry: University of Warwick Medical School.

Stickler, D (2014) *The body economic: Why austerity kills*, London: Penguin.

Stouffer, SA, Suchman, EA, DeVinney, LC, Star, SA and Williams, RM (1949) *The American soldier: Adjustment during army life*, Princeton, NJ: Princeton University Press.

Tengland, P (2013) Behavior change or empowerment: On the ethics of health promotion goals, *Health Care Analysis*, 24, 1, 24–46.

The Health Foundation (2017) *Healthy lives for people in the UK*, London: The Health Foundation.

The Herald (2014) Revealed: 20 rivers in Scotland polluted by toxic 'gender-bender' chemicals, *The Herald*, 11 May, www. heraldscotland.com/news/13159852.Revealed__20_rivers_ in_Scotland_polluted_by_toxic__gender_bender__chemicals/.

The Irish News (2016) NI Water fined £13,000 for river pollution, The Irish News, 5 November, http://www. irishnews.com/news/2016/11/05/news/ni-water-fined-13-000-for-river-pollution-770463/.

The Jakarta Conference (1997) *Leading health promotion into the 21st century*, www.who.int/healthpromotion/conferences/ previous/jakarta/declaration/en/.

The Mexico Global Conference (2000) *Fifth Global Conference on Health Promotion*, Mexico City, 5 June, www.who.int/ healthpromotion/conferences/previous/mexico/en/.

The Times (2017) 119 inmates killed themselves in gaol in 2016, *The Times*, 21 March, p 4.

Thorogood, M and Britton, A (2010) Evaluating intervention, in Thorogood, M and Coombes, Y (eds) *Evaluating health promotion: Practice and methods*, Oxford: Oxford University Press, 41–56.

Thorogood, M and Coombes, Y (eds) (2010) *Evaluating health promotion: Practice and methods*, Oxford: Oxford University Press.

Tinson, A, Ayrton, C, Barker, K, Born, TB, Aldridge, H and Kenway, P (2016) Monitoring poverty and social exclusion, *Joseph Rowntree Foundation*, www.jrf.org.uk/report/monitoring-poverty-and-social-exclusion-2016.

Tolley, K (1993) *Health promotion: How to measure cost-effectiveness*, London: Health Education Authority.

Tones, BK (1986) Health education and the ideology of health promotion: A review of alternative approaches, *Health Education Research*, 1, 3–12.

Tones, K (2001) Effectiveness in health promotion indicators and evidence, in Scott, D and Weston, R (eds) *Evaluating health promotion*, Cheltenham: Thornes, 49–74.

Tovey, M (2017) *Obesity and the public purse*, IEA discussion paper no. 80, London: Institute of Economic Affairs.

Townsend, P (1979) *Poverty in the United Kingdom*, London: Allen Lane.

Townsend, P, Phillimore, P and Beattie, A (1988) *Health and deprivation: Inequality and the North*, London: Croom Helm.

UN General Assembly (2015) *Transforming our world: the 2030 Agenda for Sustainable Development*, United Nation, https://sustainabledevelopment.un.org/post2015/transformingourworld.

Van der Knaap, P (1995) Policy evaluation and learning, *Evaluation*, 1, 2, 189–216.

Victorian Government (2008) *Measuring health promotion impacts: A guide to impact evaluation in integrated health promotion*, Victoria: Department Of Human Services.

Wallerstein, N (1992) Powerlessness, empowerment and health: Implications for health promotion programs, *Journal of Health Promotion*, 6, 3, 197–205.

Wallerstein, N (2002) Empowerment to reduce health disparities, *Scandinavian Journal of Public Health*, 30, 72 –77.

Walsh, R (2011) Lifestyle and mental health, *American Psychologist*, 66, 7, 579–92.

Wanless, D (2004) *Securing good health for the whole population*, London: HMSO.

Weale, S. (2016) Report on Speech by Nancy Devon MP, *The Guardian*, 29 April.

Wear, A (1992) Making sense of health and the environment in early modern England, in Wear, A (ed) *Medicine in society: Historical essays*, Cambridge: Cambridge University Press.

Webber, M (2006) *Health needs assessment 2006: Nutrition and obesity*, Health Information Analysis Team NPHS (National Population Health Survey).

Webster, C (1990) *The Victorian public health legacy: A challenge to the future*, London: Public Health Alliance.

Weiss, C (1972) *Evaluation research*, New Jersey, NJ: Englewood Cliffs.

Whitehead, M (1992) The concepts and principles of equity and health, *International Journal of Health Services*, 22, 3, 429–46.

WHO (World Health Organization) (1946) *Constitution: Basic Documents,* Geneva: WHO.

WHO (1977) Achieving health for all: World Health report 1998: who/int/whr/1998.

WHO (1981) *Global strategy for health for all by the year 2000*, Geneva: WHO.

WHO (1984) *Health promotion: A World Health Organization document on the concepts and principles*, Copenhagen: WHO.

WHO (1986) *The Ottawa Charter for Health Promotion: First International Conference on Health Promotion*, 21 November, Copenhagen, www.who.int/healthpromotion/conferences/previous/ottawa/en/index1.html.

WHO (1998a) *Health for all for the 21st century*, Geneva: WHO.

WHO (1998b) *Health promotion evaluation: Recommendations to policy makers – Report of the working group on health promotion evaluation*, EUR/ICP/VST 050103, Copenhagen: WHO/EURO.

WHO (2002) *Reducing risks, promoting healthy life,* Geneva: World Health Organization.

WHO (2005) *Bangkok Charter for Health Promotion in a Globalized World*, Bangkok: WHO, www.who.int/healthpromotion/ conferences/6gchp/bangkok_charter/en/.

WHO (2007) *Civil Society report: Commission on social determinants of health*, Geneva: World Health Organization.

WHO (2008) *A strategy for health promotion in the Eastern Mediterranean region 2006–2013*, http://applications.emro.who. int/dsaf/dsa794.pdf.

WHO (2009a) *Milestones in health promotion: Statements from global conferences*, Geneva: WHO.

WHO (2009b) *Nairobi call to action*, Geneva: WHO.

WHO (2009c) *World health statistics*, Geneva: World Health Organization.

WHO (2016a) *Health promotion 2016*, Shanghai: WHO and National Health and Family Planning Commission of China.

WHO (2016b) *What is health promotion?* www.who.int/features/ qa/health-promotion/en.

WHO (2017) *Monitoring health for the sustainable development goals*, Geneva: WHO, www.who.int/gho/publications/ world_health_statistics/2017/en.

WHO Commission (2008) *Closing the gap in a generation*, Geneva: WHO.

WHO European Region (1999) *Health 2: The health policy framework for the WHO European Region*, Copenhagen: WHO Regional Office for Europe.

WHO European Regional Office (2010) *A changing Europe*, www.euro.who.int.

WHO Regional Office for Europe (1998) *Health for all policy framework*, Copenhagen: World Health Organization.

WHO Regional Office for Africa (2013) *Health promotion strategy for the African region*, Brazzaville, Congo: WHO.

WHO SE Asia Regional Office (2008) *Regional strategy for health promotion in SE Asia*, New Delhi: WHO.

Wilkinson, RG (1996) *Unhealthy societies: The affliction of inequality*, London: Routledge.

Wilkinson, RG (ed) (2003) *Social determinants of health: The solid facts*, Copenhagen: WHO Regional Office for Europe.

Williams, A (1992) Cost-effectiveness analysis: Is it ethical? *Journal of Medical Ethics*, 18, 7–11.

Williams, A (1993) Speech at the Health Outcomes Conference, 16 September 1993, quoted in MacClachan, R and Glasman, D, A case of myth management, *Health Service Journal*, 103, 5370, 12–13.

Winter, JM (1980) Military fitness and civilian health in Britain during the First World War, *Journal of Contemporary History*, 15, 211–44.

Wohl, AS (1984) *Endangered lives: Public health in Victorian Britain*, London: Unwin Methuen.

Wonderling, D and Karnon, J (2010) Economic evaluation of health promotion programmes, in Thorogood, M and Coombes, Y (eds) *Evaluating health promotion: Practice and methods*, 70–83, Oxford: Oxford University Press.

Woodall, J (2007) Barriers to positive mental health in a Young Offenders Institution: a quantitative study, *Health Education Journal*, 66, 132, 132–40.

Woodall, J, Raine, G, South, J and Warwick-Booth, L (2010) *Empowerment, health and well-being: Evidence review*, Leeds: Leeds Metropolitan University.

World Economic Forum (2016) *These are the 5 health challenges facing Latin America*, www.weforum.org/agenda/2016/06/these-are-the-5-health-challenges-facing-latin-america/.

Young Report (2010) *Common sense, common safety*, London: HM Government.

Zechmeister, I, Kilian, R and McDaid, D (2008) Is it worth investing in mental health promotion and prevention of mental illness? A systematic review of the evidence from economic evaluation, *BioMedCentral Public Health*, 8, 20, https://bmcpublichealth.biomedcentral.com/articles/10.1186/1471-2458-8-20.

Index